T0129738

REVIVE

The Wellness, Fitness and
Beauty Program to
Vibrant Health

D. McCants-Reed

WESTBOW
PRESS®
A DIVISION OF THOMAS NELSON
& ZONDERVAN

WestBow Press books may be ordered through booksellers or by contacting:

WestBow Press
A Division of Thomas Nelson & Zondervan
1663 Liberty Drive
Bloomington, IN 47403
www.westbowpress.com
1 (866) 928-1240

ISBN: 978-1-9736-4332-6 (sc)
ISBN: 978-1-9736-4331-9 (hc)
ISBN: 978-1-9736-4333-3 (e)

Library of Congress Control Number: 2018912477

Print information available on the last page.

WestBow Press rev. date: 11/27/2018

Contents

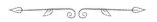

What are people saying about the Revive Program?

> Thank you for the opportunity to participate in the Revive Program. It was life changing and I don't say that lightly. I lost a total of thirty pounds during your seven-week program. I believe the Bible study you've included in the Revive Program is a huge part of why the program is so successful. Anyone who believe that their body is the temple where God dwells will find the Bible study portion of this program to be the map to total success. I did. My life will never be the same. I am slimmer, I look better, and I am healthier than I have ever been.
>
> —Joe Ann Jones, Corona CA

> I joined the Revive Wellness Program in January 2004 after being convicted in my spirit to take better care of my body. By the time I completed the program, I'd lost nine pounds, and was able to significantly reduce medication for high blood pressure and acid reflux. Most importantly, the information gained throughout the program will be with me for life.
>
> —Ron Hamilton, Cerritos, CA

> The Revive Program increased my knowledge of what it takes to be spiritually and physically well.
>
> —Jimi Roberson, Hacienda Heights, CA

> The Revive Program was a life changing opportunity. I changed my eating habits in a short period of time and it was effective. I saw the proof in the reduction of my body weight. I lost seventeen pounds.
>
> —Dennis Birthwright, Artesia, CA

I enjoyed the program. I especially like that the program incorporates mind, body, and spirit. The Bible study helps to keep you focused.

—Shirley Brown, Los Angeles, CA

My family and I together lost over two hundred pounds in the Revive Program, but for us the Bible study really helped us stay focused on the importance of staying on track, and the fellowship allowed us to help each other as we progressed through the journey of a healthy lifestyle.

—Tonya Spurling, Long Beach, CA

Preface

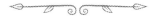

Revive: The Wellness, Fitness, and Beauty Program began one night in 1998. It was a simple telephone conversation between Kathy Dockery, the founder of Christian Business & Professional Women's Ministries, and me. We made general comments about our health, mostly complaining about being tired or too busy and, in general, the need to eat better.

Kathy asked a question, not really thinking that it would explode into anything. She said, "How did Jesus do it?"

I said, "Do what?"

She said, "How did Jesus stay healthy and fit and do God's work all at the same time?"

After we thought about it, we came up with really simple stuff. He ate healthy, meditated on the word of God, developed a strong relationship with God, and he walked a lot.

What did Jesus eat? The Bible says he ate fresh fruit, fish, bread, and meat, and the meat was certainly not prepared the way most of us eat it today. It appears that it was cooked over an open fire, and the fat dripped off. He drank lots of water, and he walked almost everywhere he traveled. He even climbed mountains.

As a result of this, we decided that we wanted to be more like Jesus in every area of our lives, and it was from this premise that Revive was born. That conversation took place twenty years ago, and the Revive Program continues to change the lives of people every day.

Acknowledgments

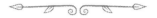

In everything that I do, my first thanks and praise is always to God. Second, I would like to thank the many friends and participants for their support and encouragement throughout the years: my sister Jimi Roberson; my dear friends, Kathy Dockery and Christian Business and Professional Women's Ministries, and Joe Ann Jones; Bishop Edward Smith and Lady Vanessa of Zoe Christian Fellowship of Whittier, Whittier, California, for their support and for giving me a platform; and the rest of the Zoe family.

My Story

Although the concept of the Revive Wellness, Fitness, and Beauty Program was developed as a result of a conversation with a dear friend, I, at the same time, was struggling with my own personal health issues. I was diagnosed in 1995 with hypothyroidism and placed on medication.

In the following year I was diagnosed with high cholesterol. My doctor at the time, again wanted to prescribe medication.

I said, "Enough is enough. There has got to be another way." I then asked, "Is there an alternative?"

My doctor suggested, with no guarantees, a change in diet and exercise. In essence, he was saying that I had to stop eating the way I was eating and move. This prompted me to make extensive changes in my life. Armed with the knowledge that I could possibly eliminate the prescribed medication, I immersed myself in research about healthy eating, wellness, and fitness. After much prayer, trial, and error, I developed a plan that worked for me.

As a result of changes in my diet, eating habits, and a regimen of regular exercise and much prayer, I no longer take medicine for hypothyroidism, and my cholesterol is manageable. The Revive Program is not a diet plan. It's a way of life. As a result of the development of the program, and my personal testimony, the Revive Wellness, Fitness and Beauty Program has helped others facing similar health challenges make necessary lifestyle changes. The path to health and wellness is straightforward. How you chose to implement it makes the difference.

Caution: Before starting this program or any lifestyle change, it's recommended that you consult your physician, especially if you're under a doctor's care, taking medication or have any medical condition that may be affected by any types of food or food allergies. Also, note the disclaimer at the beginning of this book.

Program Overview

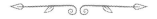

The Revive Wellness, Fitness, and Beauty Program is a seven-week program designed to help established a healthy way of life based on Christian principles. The entire seven-week program is geared toward health and wellness and achieving spiritual growth. The program is not designed with a focus on weight loss. However, this will occur if you follow the plan. It's simply a way of life that provides knowledge to a healthy rejuvenating lifestyle.

The objective of the program is to help promote wellness when you follow a nutritional diet and exercise plan. This plan may preserve our health, provide a safe program for weight loss, provide spiritual growth, sharpen our minds, and possibly slow aging.

The program requires a seven-week commitment, just forty-nine days. It's specifically designed for those men and women who have a sincere desire to improve their overall health. The program consists of small steps that build in increments weekly until, at the completion of the program, participants will have laid the foundation for healthy living.

The program is biblically based and the premier scripture can be found in Proverbs 2:10–11: "When wisdom enters your heart, and knowledge is pleasant to your soul, discretion will preserve you; understanding will keep you." When you've learned something, you have the power to choose that which will keep you in perfect health, because it's the will of God that we prosper and be in good health.

The program will also cover what I discovered are the seven mental secrets to vibrant health. Each of these seven secrets lay the foundation for the seven weekly Bible lessons, coupled with the seven weekly wellness sessions. The program is challenging, yet enjoyable, and those who wish to participate in it must be motivated to make a complete break with their lifelong or old way of living, concerning food, exercise, and beauty habits. If you're serious about making a change, do so with 100 percent of your effort.

The material required to begin and complete the program is this book (which can also function as your workbook) and your Bible. The book is divided into four parts: the Revive Wellness Program and summary guide, the Revive Bible lessons, recipes for each week, and Bible study discussions. The book also offers separate note pages for each week for your personal reflections at the end of each chapter. The weekly wellness program and Bible lessons are housed together in each chapter for continuity.

As you begin this program, just know that this program is personal to you. It's all about you and God and no one else. Whatever you write in your book are your personal thoughts, needs, wishes, or desires. This is one of the reasons that I suggest that you don't share or duplicate your materials. Again, before starting this program or any lifestyle change, it's recommended that you consult your physician, especially if you're under a doctor's care, taking medication, or have any medical condition that may be affected by any types of food or food allergies. Also, note the disclaimer at the beginning of this book.

Prior to beginning week one, take a photo or yourself. Next, weigh yourself, then record your weight on the note page found at the end of week one in this book. Next, take a tape measure and measure your chest area, waist, and hips. Record your measurements on the same page and attach your photo. This will allow you to track your progress and will also give you a before and after view of your success at the end of the program.

Participants may embark on this journey individually or in a group. If in a group setting you'll meet once a week for one hour, select a partner and receive instruction and guidance from the program facilitator. During this hour, the group will have prayer, weekly Bible study discussion, wellness program instructions, support from mentoring partners, fitness and beauty tips, and celebrate victories. Yes, to answer your question, this can all be done in one hour. Single or individual program participants will follow the layout and instructions given weekly in each chapter. You, the participant, can decide how much of this program you want to maintain on a permanent basis. The overall program consists of five areas: wellness, fitness, beauty (skin care), mentoring, and spiritual growth. Each area consists of the following:

1. Wellness—Each week, participants are provided with a basic nutrition guide that focus on a specific nutritional step designed for the week. This step is to be added and continued throughout the program.

2. Fitness—Participants, during the first weeks, will select fitness activities of their choice to engage in throughout the program. It can be anything, such as walking, running, swimming, or playing tennis, but you must select something. This does not mean that you're limited to that activity and can't engage in other activities. As you grow each week, feel free to broaden your horizon.

3. Beauty (Skin Care)—Each participant is encouraged to engage in a healthy daily skin-care routine to assist with skin-care maintenance and protection. Beauty tips will be given in each session if participating as a group.

4. Mentoring—If beginning the program with a partner or in a group, participants are encouraged in the first week to identify a partner within the group to assist in the participant's success. The purpose here is to provide support and develop relationships.

5. Spiritual Growth—This is the weekly Bible lesson. Each participant will complete the assigned Bible lesson to utilize as a self-study for the week. If meeting as a group, the Bible lesson and discussion will be a part of the week's group session.

The Seven Mental Secrets to Vibrant Health

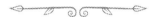

As participants of the program, you'll learn and apply the seven mental secrets to vibrant health from a biblical perspective, as each mental secret is the central focus of the weekly Bible lesson. To each participant, I freely and joyfully share the following:

The seven mental secrets to vibrant health

1. Believe that you can do it. (Mark 9:23)
2. Make an unyielding commitment (Romans 12:1, Proverbs 16:3)
3. Set realistic goals. (Luke 14:28–30)
4. Visualize success. (Habakkuk 2:2–3)
5. Hold yourself accountable (Genesis 3:12)
6. Maintain a record. (Proverbs 27:23)
7. Rebound and learn from mistakes. (2 Peter 1:2–3, 8–9)

Mental Secret Number One—Believe that you can do it. "Jesus said unto him; If thou canst believe. All things are possible to him that believeth" (Mark 9:23). A belief is an indisputable version of that which we hold to be true or false. So if you want to live a healthy lifestyle, and you believe that you can do it, you must be constant and vigilant in holding this belief strongly in your mind, because it's important that you respond to your inner most thoughts with the word of God. The Bible says, "Let this mind be in you which was also in Christ Jesus" (Philippians 2:5). Believe in yourself and have faith in your abilities.

Meditate on Philippians 4:13. "I can do all things through Christ Jesus which strengthen me."

Mental Secret Number Two—Make a firm commitment. "Commit thy works unto the Lord and thy thoughts shall be established" (Proverbs 16:3). Commitment means to take on an obligation; it means to trust and empower. We as Christians have a duty to embrace our health and well-being so that we may be fit to do God's work. Whatever you do, do it all for God's glory. This includes your health and eating habits. Commit your health to the Lord, and he will empower you to do his work. I once saw a sign that read, "Anything that you cannot commit to will go away." If you can't commit to your health, it, too, will go away.

Mental Secret Number Three—Set realistic goals. "For which of you intending to build a tower, sitteth not down first, and counteth the cost, whether he have sufficient to finish it. Lest haply, after, he hath laid the foundation, and is not able to finish it. All that behold it begin to mock him saying, this man began to build and was not able to finish" (Luke 14: 28–30). Often, people set a goal that's unrealistic. This sometimes can be the downfall of any process. So, in establishing or setting your goals for this program, make sure that they are attainable. If losing fifteen pounds in seven weeks is your goal, this is attainable. If reading the Bible one hour a day is your goal or praying one hour a day or walking one hour a day is your goal, this also is attainable. Start with small steps and build. Your goals are personal to you and not to others. Take a few minutes now and set your goal for this program. Focus in the areas of health, wellness, and spiritual growth. What do you want to accomplish in seven weeks? What do you want to accomplish in six months? What do you want to accomplish for the rest of your life, in every area of your life? Write your thoughts and goals in the note section of your book. In our attempts to become better Christians, we grow a little at a time. God does not expect us to be perfect, so let's take this walk one step at a time. You did not develop bad eating habits overnight, so you can't change them overnight. It's a process as everything else is in our life.

Mental Secrets Number Four—Visualize success. "And the Lord answered me and said, write the vision and make it plain upon the tables that he may run that readeth it, for the vision is yet for an appointed time, but at the end, it shall speak and not lie; though it may tarry, wait for it, because it will surely come, it will not tarry" (Habakkuk 2:2–3). If you can visualize it, you can achieve it with God's help. So, when you begin this program, see yourself the way you want to be, then start to work toward the vision. You may want to start, by finding a picture of yourself, or your favorite dress or pants that you can no longer wear. Put it in an area that you'll see daily for motivation. You may also at this time start a vision board.

Mental Secret Number Five—Hold yourself accountable. "And the man said, the woman whom thou gavest to be with me, she gave me of the tree and I did eat" (Genesis 3:12). Here as you can see, Adam is playing the blame game. We have to stop playing the blame game. We have to stop blaming others for our lack of success. In order to be successful in this program, you must take responsibility for you own actions. So whatever your excuses are, take time now to speak them into a paper bag, tie it up, and then throw it in the garbage container outside of your house. Don't bring it back into your house by speaking the same excuses or other excuses in existing, because it's toxic. It's garbage. I want you to stop and take a minute and really visualize what is placed in garbage containers. Don't just look on the surface, go to the middle, then to the bottom. Okay. Do you want to bring this back into your house? That's what you're doing when you continue to make excuses that lead to the road of nothingness. "Being confident of this very thing, that he which hath begun a good work in you will perform it until the day of Jesus" (Philippians 1:6).

Mental Secret Number Six—Maintain a record. "Be thou diligent to know the state of thy flocks and look well to thy heard" (Proverbs 27:23). Record your progress weekly from beginning to end. You may use the note section in your book, or you can use a journal to track your journey. Keep it by your bed for easy access. Write praises and thanks to God for allowing you to come this far.

Mental Secret Number Seven—Rebound and learn from your mistakes. In the Bible, 2 Peter 1:2–3 speaks about the knowledge of God and all things that apply to life through the knowledge of God. These are the things we learn and acquire through trial and error. "For if these things be in you, and abound, they make you that ye shall neither be barren nor unfruitful in the knowledge of our Lord Jesus Christ" (2 Peter 1:8). Knowledge is power. What you'll learn in this program will lay the foundation for the rest of your life. If you fall off the wagon one day, slip and eat the wrong thing, get up and get back on, because you'll get where you're going, if you keep going in the right direction.

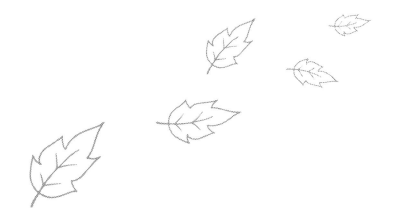

Fasting and Cleansing

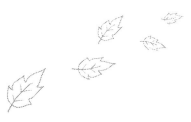

Wellness: Week One

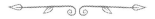

Program Commencement

Make a notation on your calendars, and in seven short weeks (or forty-nine days from today), you may, depending on how well you follow the program, look radiant, feel energized, be healthier and mentally alert. Really: you'll feel revived.

Week One

If you haven't already, take a photo or yourself. Next, weigh yourself and then record your weight on the note page found at the end of week one in this book. Next, take a tape measure, and measure your chest area, waist, and hips. Record your measurements on the same page and attach your photo. Weigh yourself at the end of week one. Don't weigh yourself again until the end of the program. This week begins with fasting and cleansing. During week one, for example, I complete a natural detox or an herbal colon cleanse for three to five days. Again, I also ask that you review the disclaimer located at the beginning of this book and again at the end of this section. I suggest that you consult your physician before you begin this program or any other program that's health-related.

In *Candida: A Natural Approach,* authors Shirley Trickett and Karen Brody explain that a toxic colon is a major factor in or cause of chronic ill health. They further illustrate that the colon is the main organ responsible for ridding the body of toxic waste, and if this is functioning poorly (for example, due to diet, stress, drugs, chemicals, or other substances), it produces a poisonous or toxic residue along the lining of the colon that irritates or inflames the colon. When the colon is inflamed, this poison is circulated via your blood through the lymphatic system.

Don't panic, and don't think you can cure this problem with one cleansing. You can't, but it's a beginning—along with everything else you'll be doing in this program. In a 2017 interview, naturopath Dr. Marilyn Mitchell, of Nature's Raw Truth explained that; even though the human body has the natural ability to detoxify itself, the objective of a natural detoxing system is to eliminate toxic or poisonous residue stored in the body that affects our vital organs. She further indicated that if you can work on removing the toxins from your body, followed by nourishing it with healthy nutrients, this may help to protect you from disease and chronic illness, resulting in good health.

Think about the buildup of toxicity in your system this way: You have only one pot to cook all of your food, and there are no exceptions. As you cook in this same pot for years and years, cleaning it as best as you can after each use, you still have residue remaining in the pot. This residue is caked in and around all areas of the pot and is incorporated into each new use thereafter, causing contamination. This goes throughout your body, as the contaminated food is eaten and digested.

What do you think is happening in your body, and how can you stop the contamination? One way to remedy this is to remove the toxins from your body through a cleanse. That's what detoxing does. I don't suggest or believe in harsh laxatives. I personally find that an all-natural detox herbal cleanser works better for me because it's natural and tends to work better with my body. I personally prefer the Nature's Raw Truth Detox System. Here again, it's suggested that you consult your physician on what is best for you.

Fasting

The next step is fasting. We call week one a fast because you'll be giving up almost everything that you normally eat for the next seven days. During the next seven days, you'll eat nothing but fresh fruits and vegetables. If you need to eat bread or a cracker to take your medication, continue to do so.

Vitamins

The next thing that you may do is add a vitamin supplement. If you take a vitamin supplement, continue to do so. Prior to beginning this journey, the word *vitamin* was foreign to me. After beginning the program, I realized how important it is that my body receive the necessary nutrients to function effectively. *The American Medical Association Family Medical Guide* alerts us that although food is the best source of nutrients, most doctors now recommend that most people take a daily multivitamin/mineral supplement to ensure that they get all of the essential nutrients.

In *Vitamania: Our Obsessive Quest for Nutritional Perfection*, Catherine Price points out that vitamins constitute one of several categories of nutrients necessary for normal body growth, maintenance, and tissue repair. In addition, in the *Complete Food & Nutrition Guide* published by the Academy of Nutrition and Dietetics, Roberta L. Duyff lets us know that vitamins and minerals are key to every process that takes place in our bodies. In assessing the benefits of vitamins, it's clear that they are essential and contribute to good health. Throughout the next seven weeks, because you'll be changing your eating habits, it may be helpful to add a multivitamin to your diet. Consult your doctor to determine if this is something that you should add for daily nutrition intake.

Fruits and Vegetables

The benefits of eating fruits and vegetables are far-reaching. While growing up and through adulthood, my siblings and I were told to eat our vegetables. I grew up in the south, and fresh fruit and vegetables were plentiful, so it was a no-brainer. These things were simply part of our daily diet, but I had no idea how much these nutrients contributed to my health. In the *Complete Food & Nutrition Guide,* Duyff points out that research has shown that eating enough vegetables and fruit is associated with reduced risks of many chronic diseases, including cardiovascular disease, and may protect against some types of cancer. In "About Fruits and Vegetables," an article published on February 23, 2017, by the American Heart Association, fruits and vegetables are noted as being high in vitamins and minerals, and it appears that they have amazing benefits.

In June 2014, CNN presented a live special by the Nutrition Twins highlighting four surprising benefits of vegetables: they fight bloat, create a youthful glow, reduce stress, and protect bones. Armed with this knowledge, we can easily understand why we are constantly encouraged by the health industry to eat more fruits and vegetables. According to Brenda Watson, CNC, and Leonard Smith, MD, in *The Fiber35 Diet: Nature's Weight Loss Secret,* fruits are high in fiber and water and loaded with disease-fighting phytonutrients. With all of these built-in properties, it can be implied that fruit can be fibrous and a natural cleanser for the body. Fruits are commonly known to be rich sources of antioxidants, and they contribute to our overall good health. Because some fruits are high in sugar content, if you have food allergies or medical issues that address high glycemic intake, you may want to avoid or limit your intake of this type. Don't eat any canned or dried fruit throughout the program.

Vegetables play a major role in our overall good health. Most vegetables are powerful stimulants that serve to activate the body's metabolism, which in many ways may act to keep the body functioning effortlessly. Although fresh vegetables are preferred, you may eat frozen vegetables, but be sure to rinse the vegetables of excess ice prior to cooking. For the first three days, eat all of your vegetables raw. This means that you must wait to eat frozen vegetables unless you're making fruit-and-vegetable smoothies; then using frozen fruit is permissible. For the last four days, you may do a combination of cooked and raw.

The first three days of raw vegetables with the natural detox or colon cleanse will help your body get used to pushing the roughage through your system. For the last four days, in addition to eating raw vegetables, you may steam, grill, bake, or broil your vegetables—no frying. You may not use butter, cheese, dairy products, or heavy sauces on your vegetables during this program. You're not limited to seasonings or herbs. You may use nonstick sprays (olive and canola oils). You may use any type of salad dressings. You're not limited in the amount, but keep in mind that some dressings are high in dairy, cheeses, and calories. One of my all-time favorites is oil and vinegar. If you don't like prepared dressings, you may use a rice vinegar or simply squeeze lemon juice on your salad. Again, your dressings are a personal choice.

This week, you may eat as much as you like, as often as you like. Whenever you get hungry, have some vegetables or fruit close by. Keep in mind that you're not on a diet, so don't begin to think in this manner or limit your intake of vegetables to such a level that you're constantly hungry. You may eat any kind of vegetables, preferably fresh. You may use frozen vegetables if fresh are unavailable. If at all possible, try to avoid canned vegetables. If you're in an area where fresh vegetables are unavailable, you may use canned vegetables, but rinse and drain them thoroughly to reduce sodium intake. Remember: potatoes and corn are not vegetables and can't be a part of your first week's nutrition. These selections will be incorporated later in the program. Helpful recipes for week one can be found in the recipe section of the book.

As you prepare your plant-based foods throughout the program—and for the rest of your life—make sure to incorporate a variety of colors in your food plan, as recommended by naturopath Dr. Marilyn Mitchell of Nature's Raw Truth. She explained in our October 5, 2017, interview that plant-based foods not only add radiant color to your diet but also are rich in nutrients, as each color is attributed to a significant health benefit. She suggests that we think about the various colors of the rainbow when putting salads and stir-fry dishes together.

Preparation Tips: As you begin each week, I suggest that you purchase most of your fruits and vegetables. Clean and chop all vegetables. Separate and place in sealed air tight containers. This is a time-saving tip and allows quick and easy access when you're ready to eat. Another time-saving and helpful tip I discovered was making a pot of vegetable soup at the beginning of each week. It adds bulk and fiber and helps to curve your appetite. There is no limit to the amount of fresh fruit and vegetables you can eat this week. Eat as much as you like and as often as you like.

I know that some of you, because of time and convenience, will often purchase prepackaged salads. That's fine, but make sure that you rinse the lettuce or kale thoroughly prior to eating. If you purchase prepackage salads, the nuts, candied fruits, or croutons included are not a part of your food plan for week's one through six. The nuts may can be added in week seven. The candied or dried fruits are to be eliminated entirely.

Water

The next thing you'll do is drink water. I always knew that water was an important nutrient, but I did not fully comprehend how crucial it was to my overall health until I began my quest for a lifestyle change. Water, in my opinion, is the key to life. It's that substance that we can't live without. Water, as explained by Phyllis A. Balch in *Prescription for Nutritional Healing*, is an essential nutrient that's involved in every function of the body. The Food and Nutrition Board of the Institute of Medicine is clear that water is essential for maintaining vascular volume and serves as the medium for transport within the body by supplying nutrients and removing waste. Water appears to be crucial to our body's ability to function normally. Water, in my opinion, can be labeled a miracle worker as it can possibly help to prevent disease, dehydration, and possibly slow aging.

The amount of water a person drinks a day appears to be in question as it's based on a number of factors such as weight, age, activity, and location. Kathleen M. Zelman, MPH, RD, LD, Director of Nutrition for WebMD in an article, "The Wonders of Water," lists the recommendations as set forth by the Institute of Medicine based on total fluid intake. For women, 91 ounces or eleven-plus cups a day, and men 125 ounces or fifteen-plus cups a day.

Isadore Rosenfeld MD in *Live Now, Age Later: Proven Ways to Slow Down the Clock* clarifies the need to drink eight glasses of water a day to prevent constipation. Dr. Andrew Weil also explains in *Natural*

Health, Natural Medicine why drinking plenty of good quality water is essential to health. He recommends that we drink six to eight glasses a day of fluid that's mostly water. The Mayo Clinic in a September 2017 article, "Water How Much Should You Drink," address studies that have produced varying recommendations over the years.

The article also illustrates that our bodies depend on water to survive and drinking eight glasses a day is easy to remember and it's a reasonable goal. However, for this program in addition to any other fluids, the suggestion is the eight-glass rule. The suggestion is that you drink at least eight glasses of clear water a day. No additives other than lemon or lime, if you need it. Each glass should be eight ounces. You may drink anything else such as coffee, herbal teas, and some juices. Keep in mind that most juices contain large quantities of sugar. If you decide to drink juices or other liquids during this program, it's still suggested in addition to the juices and teas, to drink the eight glasses of water a day. You may not drink milk this first week. However, if you add milk in your coffee or tea, this is the exception. Your results depend on how well you follow the program.

Fitness

The next thing you'll do is exercise. As we are all aware, exercise plays a major role toward health and wellness. It contributes to weight loss by burning calories, accelerates slow metabolisms, strengthens muscles, and contributes to overall fitness. The *Family Medical Guide* published by the American Medical Association indicates that physical activity plays a crucial role in health. The American Heart Association also indicates that regular exercise protects against the most common disorders, including heart disease, strokes, high blood pressure, obesity, type 2 diabetes, osteoporosis, colon cancer and depression.

Exercise is an important part of this program if you want to see measurable results. I have provided a list of possible physical activities for your review. This list is not intended to be exclusive. Go to that section in the book and select an activity or any other activities that works for you. Select a physical activity that fits into your daily lifestyle, be it walking, swimming, jogging, or dancing. The minimum exercise requirement for this week is thirty minutes a day for five days. This will increase in interval each week. You must incorporate some form of physical activity to see measurable results. If you're already exercising on a regular basis, please continue. For those of you who are having a problem getting started, you may want to seek the assistance of a personal trainer or maybe join a gym. There are also numerous exercise tapes and videos available on the market that may assist you with this endeavor.

Beauty

The next thing you'll do for the next seven weeks is develop a regular skin-care routine. In our zest for good health, it's necessary that we cover all the bases. Our skin is an important factor, according to Elsie Daniels, renowned makeup artist, beauty expert, and the owner of Hollywood Faces in Artesia, California. In a January 13, 2012 interview, she explained that our skin, like any other parts of our bodies, needs to be fed and cared for on the inside and outside. This, she explained, can be done on the inside through proper nutrition and drinking sufficient amounts of water. She also indicated that this could possibly be the catalyst that contributes to a youthful glow.

For outside care, she suggests four simple steps as a daily skin-care routine:

(1) Cleanse and tone in the morning and at night.
(2) Exfoliate to remove dead and dry skin.
(3) Moisturize each morning and at night prior to sleep.
(4) Apply SPF during the day.

Most skin-care products can be found in your nearest pharmacy at a modest cost. Simply read the labels and determine what works best for you. If you have a medical plan that includes a dermatologist, make an appointment to get assistance that's personalized. I use and prefer most natural products. These tend to work best for me and my body chemistry. If you already have a routine and products that work for you, please continue.

In addition to applying the four steps above, Daniels also recommends rest and relaxation making sure to get a restful night sleep every night.

Mentoring

The next thing you'll do, if in a group setting, is select a mentoring partner within the group. After selecting your partner, let him or her know that you're happy that he or she is a part of the program and has chosen to take this journey with you. Make a personal commitment to each other to attend all sessions, complete the Bible lessons, follow the nutritional steps, and contact each other regularly for encouragement and support.

Spiritual Growth

The final thing you'll do is begin the week one Bible lesson. This section can be found after the Wellness Summary Guide for each week. You're required to answer a minimum of one to two questions daily in the Bible lesson for the next seven days. Write your answers in the space provided and meditate on the scriptures throughout the week.

During the next weekly sessions, participants, if in a group, after individually completing the Bible lesson will meet and engage in active discussion, centered upon biblical principles through the guidance and directions of the program facilitator. If you're participating as a group, discuss you answers at your next week's session. If you're completing the program individually, after completing your personal Bible lesson, review the Bible study discussion answers found and labeled in the last section of this book.

At the beginning of each week, a nutrition step is added to Wellness. Fitness is increased and a new Revive Bible lesson is assigned until program completion. For an easy reference or sequential break down of each week's activity, see the Wellness Summary Guide found at the end of each wellness segment.

Now, this is the time you put the book down and go to the market, if you haven't already done so, buy all of your fresh fruits and vegetables. Clean, prepare, and store them so that they are ready when you want them. The program starts now. Let's begin with God's speed.

Begin week one Bible lesson.

Disclaimer

The Revive Wellness, Fitness, and Beauty Program is not developed by health professionals. It is based on opinions and proven testimonials of the participants. It is strongly recommended that you consult a medical professional before you begin this or any other program that contributes to weight loss. The program, it's authors, or program administrators, or any entity associated herewith, does not provide, offer, or engage in rendering medical advice or services. The authors, publishers and any entity associated herewith disclaim any responsibility, liability or loss incurred through the use and application of this program. Discuss this information with your own health-care provider to determine what is right for you.

Medical Disclaimer

All information is intended for your general knowledge only and is not a substitute for medical advice or treatment. We can't and do not give medical advice. You should seek prompt medical care for any specific health issues and consult your physician before starting a new fitness or nutrition regiment. Should you have any health-care-related questions, please see or call your physician or health-care provider promptly. The information contained in this program is presented in summary form only and intended to provide a broad consumer understanding and knowledge of health and wellness. The information should not be considered complete and should not be used in place of a visit, call, consultation or advice of your physician or other health-care provider.

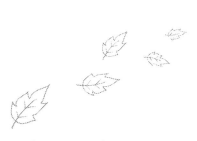

Wellness Summary Guide: Week One

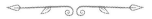

"Behold, I wish above all things that thou mayest prosper and be in good health even as thou soul prospereth" (3 John 1:2).

Wellness

Begin week one with the following steps:

1. Cleansing.
2. Take vitamin supplements (optional).
3. Fasting. Eat fresh fruits and vegetables. The first three days, eat all vegetables raw. The last four days you may eat cooked and raw vegetables. The cooked vegetables may be, steamed, grilled, baked, or broiled.
4. Drink eight glasses of water per day. Eight ounces per glass.

Fitness

"But wilt thou know, O vain man, that faith without works is dead?" (James 2:20)

1. Exercise thirty minutes per day for five days.

Beauty

1. Develop a regular skin-care routine
2. Get a restful night sleep every night.

Spiritual

1. Recharge your spirit through prayer and Bible study
2. Write a daily confession in your book

Mentoring

If beginning the program in a group, select a mentoring partner. The program facilitator will discuss exciting ways to prepare fruits and vegetables for the next seven days, the importance of fitness activities and beauty tips.

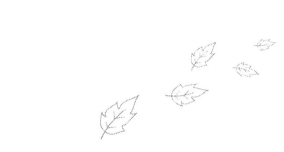

Fitness Activities

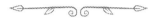

Before beginning any exercise routine, it's recommended that you consult your health-care professional. The benefits of any exercise program depend on commitment, discipline, and consistency. The following is simply a list of exercise options that you may decide to engage in. It's not intended to be inclusive.

Aerobic exercise
Bike riding
Cycling
Dancing
Golf
Handball
Roller skating
Running
Skiing
Swimming
Tennis
Treadmill
Yoga
Walking

Revive Program Notes

_____

_____

_____

_____

_____

_____

_____

_____

_____

_____

_____

_____

_____

_____

_____

_____

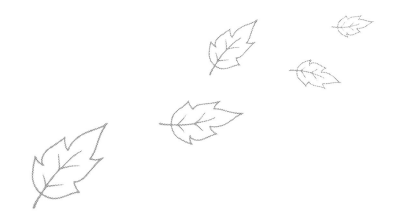

Revive Bible Lesson

Fasting and Cleansing

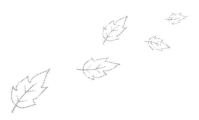

Revive Bible Lesson: Week One

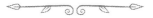

Mental Secret Number One: Believe that you can do it.

"Jesus said unto him. If thou canst believe, all things are possible to him that believeth" (Mark 9:23).

Bible Lesson One
Time: Fifteen minutes

Study Questions

1.1. What does fasting mean to you?

1.2. What does Isaiah 58:6-8 tell us about fasting? Explain its meaning and how it relates to your definition of fasting.

1.3. Why do you think it's necessary to cleanse your body to begin this program? After writing your answers, read Colossians 3:9–10, Romans 6:6. Meditate on 1 Corinthians 3:16–17.

1.4. Why is it necessary to have the right mind-set to begin this program? Read Proverbs 23:7. What does this mean to you?

1.5. How does Mark 9:23 apply to you in relations to this program?

1.6. Read and meditate on Philippians 4:13 and 2 Samuel 22:33.

Revive Program Notes

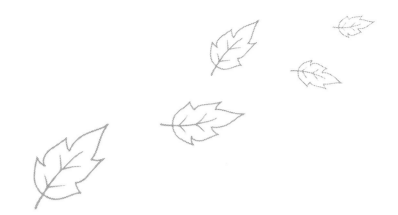

Commitment and Time Management

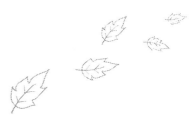

Wellness: Week Two

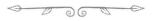

Congratulations! You've completed week one which is possibly the most difficult week of this journey. If you're still up for the challenge, let's have some fun as we travel this path of wellness, fitness, and beauty through the grace of God.

This week, you'll continue taking a vitamin supplement (optional) and drinking eight glasses of water per day (eight ounces per glass). You'll also continue eating fruits and vegetables; however, I will define the portions for each. According to the 2015–2020 Dietary Guidelines for Americans, you should consume between five to thirteen servings of fruit and vegetables a day. This, however, depends on your caloric level. The calories should be divided somewhat equally between the fruits and vegetables.

For fruit, the 2015–2020 Dietary Guidelines for Americans recommendation is two cups. That's equal to four servings a day. A serving is equivalent to one-half cup, but remember: an apple a day keeps the doctor away. Because some fruits are higher in sugar content than others, do your research and be selective. You're probably thinking, that's too much fruit, but you'll be amazed at how much fruit you eat in a day. Here's a tip. How many of you like smoothies? Simply put a small mixture of your favorite fruit in a high-speed blender, or food processor with water. Add kale or spinach, blend, and enjoy. You can also juice your fresh fruit or simply eat as a snack.

Vegetables are essential for good health. Robert Kowalski in *The New 8-Week Cholesterol Cure* states that "we should eat at least five servings of vegetables a day, preferably seven or even nine." The 2015–2020 Dietary

Guidelines for Americans suggests that you eat a minimum of five to eight servings of vegetables a day. Remember: a serving is equivalent to one-half cup, so if you eat a large salad every day, in most cases, you've eaten at best, the minimum requirement, but for this week you'll more than likely eat more than the eight servings suggested.

In order to provide and maintain a balance diet, we need to eat three kinds of nutrients—carbohydrates, fats, and proteins. In researching these areas, I discovered a plethora of information. In a 2014 review, "Balancing Carbs, Proteins, and Fats," Karen Hanson, a registered dietarian for Kaiser Permanente of Washington, DC, indicates these nutrients contain calories that your body use for energy, and 12 to 20 percent of your total daily calories should come from proteins. Sources of proteins as listed by the US Department of Agriculture 2015–2020 Dietary Guide for Americans can be found in meat, poultry, seafood, dairy, plant foods, such as beans and peas, nuts and seeds, eggs and vegetables.

The second type of nutrient are fats. These nutrients give the body energy according to Ms. Hanson, and 30 percent of total daily calories should come from fat. Carbohydrates another nutrient are the major sources of energy for the body, and I promise that, during this program, we will eat all three of the nutrients discussed above, but for this week, we will add just one, protein.

Proteins for this program can be in the form of meat or plants, such as beans or legumes. You can add this for lunch or dinner. For meat protein, I suggest only fresh fish and poultry. The American Diabetes Association, in their 2018 review, "Food and Portion Size," clarifies the serving size for meat. The serving size is about the size of the palm of your hand. The remaining space on your plate should be filled this week with vegetables. The meat can be baked, broiled, or grilled. Don't use butter, margarine, spreads or sauces. You may use your favorite spice or any spices of choice. If eating plant foods as your protein and you chose to use canned beans, make sure to rinse them thoroughly to reduce sodium intake. If you chose to eat meat, that's your protein. If you chose beans, that's your protein. Don't eat them together this week. Only one of them. Revisit portion size if unsure. There is no limitation on your servings of vegetables, but your portion size of meat proteins is set above for each day. Please, if at all possible, try not to go over the amount suggested.

Time-Saving Quick Tips for the Week

1. Plan all meals at the beginning of each week, then go to the market.
2. Make a big pot of fresh vegetable soup at the beginning of the week. (See recipe section for quick vegetable soup.)
3. Purchase all fruits and vegetables at the beginning of each week. Clean and cut all fruits and vegetables and store in separate tightly sealed containers.

Fitness—This week instead of exercising for thirty minutes, you'll increase your exercise routine to forty-five minutes per day for five days. If you decide to do more, that's great. A helpful tip is to plan a set time each day for exercise. If you can, try making it a social event by scheduling it with your mentoring partner or a friend.

You'll continue your skin-care routine and get a good night's sleep. Make time to check in with your mentoring partner.

Begin week two Revive Bible lesson.

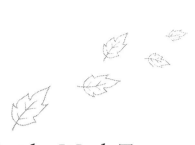

Wellness Summary Guide: Week Two

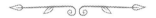

Welcome to week two.

Wellness

Begin week two with the following steps:

1. Continue taking vitamin supplements (optional).
2. Eat a minimum of three to four servings of fresh fruit daily.
3. Eat a minimum of five to eight servings of different vegetables a day.
4. Drink eight glasses of water per day. Eight ounces per glass.
5. Eat one serving of protein (fresh fish or poultry) or two servings of plant protein each day. If you chose to eat meat that's your protein. If you chose beans, that's your protein. Don't eat them together this week. Only one of them. Revisit portion size if unsure. There is no limit on your servings of vegetables, but your portion size of meat proteins is set each day. If you're a vegetarian, you may use other protein sources, but no dairy.

Fitness

1. Exercise forty-five minutes a day for five days.

Beauty

1. Continue a complete skin-care routine.
2. Continue getting a good night's sleep. If you're having a problem sleeping, consider drinking calming herbal teas.

Spiritual

1. Recharge your spirit through prayer and weekly Bible study.
2. Write a daily confession in your book.

Mentoring

1. Take a minute to make a call to encourage and support your mentoring partner.

Revive Program Notes

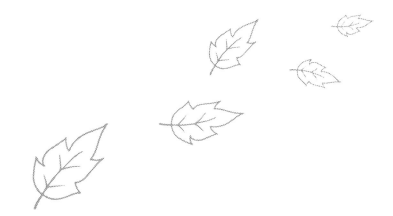

Revive Bible Lesson

Commitment and Time Management

Revive Bible Lesson: Week Two

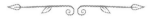

Mental Secret Number Two: Make an unyielding commitment.

"I beseech you therefore, brethren, by the mercies of God, that ye present your bodies a living sacrifice, holy, acceptable unto God, which is your reasonable service" (Romans 12:1).

"Commit thy works unto the Lord, and thy thoughts shall be established" (Proverbs 16:3).

Mental Secret Number Three: Set realistic goals.

"For which of you, intending to build a tower, sitteth not down first, and counteth the cost, whether he have sufficient to finish it? Lest haply, after he hath laid the foundation, and is not able to finish it, all that behold it begin to mock him, saying, this man begins to build and was not able to finish" (Luke 14:28–30).

Bible Lesson Two
Time: Fifteen minutes

Study Questions

2.1. In your own words write what you think it means to make a commitment.

2.2. What choices have you made concerning your commitment to Jesus?

2.3. What choices have you made concerning your commitment to this program? Think on Proverbs 16:3 as you contemplate this answer.

2.4. What does Psalm 37:5 say about commitment?

2.5. Have you set your goal for this program? Is it realistic? Write your answer, then read Luke 14:28–30. What does this scripture mean to you?

2.6. Meditate on Ecclesiastics 3:1–9 and 2 Samuel 22:33.

Revive Program Notes

_____

_____

_____

_____

_____

_____

_____

_____

_____

_____

_____

_____

_____

_____

_____

_____

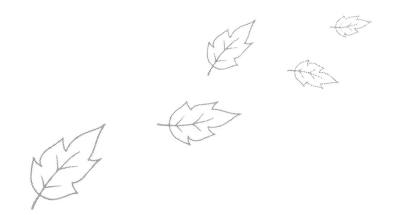

Vision, Change, and Transformation

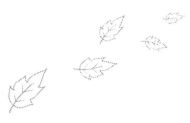

Wellness: Week Three

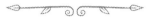

You're all awesome. You've made it to week three. May the grace of God continue to shine upon you as we travel this path, so that you may reap the fruits of your labor in due season.

How do you feel? Are you seeing results? Are you spending more time in prayer? Some of you may not be noticing a loss of pounds at this stage, but you may be experiencing a significant loss in body inches. You may find that your clothes are getting looser, but the weight is the same or slightly lower. If this is happening to you, maybe you're what I call an incher. You'll see results faster with a loss in body inches. The weight or the pounds will follow. Just keep going.

As you continue the program, think about what else is changing in your life, not just with your weight. Are you experiencing change or growth in any other areas? I strongly believe that if you can control your eating habits you can control anything else in your life that's out of control. Write your thoughts in your Revive book or start your personal journal.

Let's get started on week three. For your nutritional intake, this week you'll do everything that you were doing for the last two weeks, but we will add another nutritional step. You'll begin week three by continuing to take a vitamin supplement (optional). You'll continue to eat a minimum of three to four servings of fruit daily. You'll continue to eat a minimum of five to eight servings of different vegetables a day. (Each serving of both fruit and vegetables should be at least 1/2 cup.) You'll continue to drink eight glasses of water per day. Eight ounces each. You'll continue to eat protein daily. This may be a meat serving of fresh fish, or poultry or two servings of plant foods such as legumes.

In addition to all of the above, you'll add carbohydrates this week. Carbohydrates are types of food sources that provide energy for the body and, according to the 2015–2020 Dietary Guidelines for Americans are a part of a helpful diet. Therefore, it's important to choose carbohydrates wisely.

There are two types of carbohydrates: simple carbohydrates and complex carbohydrates. Because this area is so crucial, I feel that it's really important that you know the difference between the two and the impact that each has on your body. Like most people, prior to making a lifestyle change, I was always on the go and often made fast foods and junk food a major part of my diet. I loved any and most foods that were fried. My daily diet consisted of mostly food items such as white rice, pasta, white breads, white potatoes, pizza, processed foods, pastries, sodas, and juice, because it was fast easy and taste good.

As I explored my quest for health and a complete lifestyle change, I discovered that what I was eating was contributing to my ill health and possibly to an early demise. Susan A. Balch in *Prescription for Nutritional Healing* makes plain that most simple carbohydrates, sometimes called simple sugars, raise blood sugar levels more than complex ones, and eating foods high in glycemic index can lead to obesity, heart disease, and diabetes. Some examples she explains are your fruit juices, candy, table sugar, corn syrup, all baked goods and pasta made with white flour, white rice, sodas, most packaged cereals, and snacks or junk food. These carbohydrates appear to be sugar, and most foods that sugar is added to.

When you eat these simple carbohydrates, according to Dr. Marilyn Mitchell of Nature's Raw Truth, they cause a surge in your blood sugar, which contributes to food cravings and constant hunger. When this happens, you tend to eat more, and as you eat more, you tend to gain weight. This she indicates can contribute to ill health and speed up the aging process.

The second type of carbohydrate is complex carbohydrates. The American Cancer Society Nutritional Guidelines in Eat Healthy and

Get Active recommends avoiding processed and refined carbohydrates in favor of complex ones, as much as possible. According to the American Cancer Society in their April 6, 2017 review, "Good for You Carbohydrates," complex carbohydrates are digested more slowly and supply a lower steadier release of glucose into the blood stream and they are high in nutrients and contain good amounts of vitamins, minerals, and fiber. Complex carbohydrates, according to numerous sources, including the 2015–2020 Dietary Guide for Americans, are such things as fruits, vegetables, nuts and seeds, multigrain bread, brown rice, and legumes, which are dried beans such as lentils and black beans.

In the 2017 review "Grains and Starchy Vegetables" published by the American Diabetes Association, starchy vegetables are potatoes, corn, and peas. The review also cautions that although these foods can be a part of a healthy diet, they do raise blood glucose. However, we should try to include them into several meals per week. So, for this week and the rest of the program you may add, but limit the amount of starchy vegetables such as corn, peas, and potatoes to no more than three to four servings weekly. One serving equals to one ear of fresh or frozen corn or one medium potato. (Exceptions for vegetarians.)

Wheat and grains are contained in most breads and can cause a rise in your blood sugar. Let's look at serving size. For breads, limit the amount to two servings a day. One serving is equal to one slice of bread. So, in essence if you're having a sandwich or hamburger you've eaten your serving of bread for the day. Your bread choices are whole grain, wheat bread, sprouted bread, or flourless breads. So, for the rest of this program and for the rest of your life, keep in mind that this is a lifestyle change. You'll eliminate white rice, white pasta, white bread, sugary cereals, snacks, and junk foods from your diet. You'll replace your bread choices with whole grains, wheat, sprouted, or flourless breads as indicated above. You can find these products in most health food stores, and they cost no more than the breads in major super markets.

This is an example thus far of what a typical day now looks on the Revive Program:

Breakfast: Serving of oatmeal (no butter or white sugar), or you can have an egg or vegetable omelet cooked with nonstick spray, and a serving of fresh fruit, or a fruit-and-vegetable smoothie. Drink water. In addition, you may also drink coffee or tea.

Snack: Serving of fruit or vegetables and water.

Lunch: Large colorful salad with an array of vegetables as you continue to drink water throughout the day.

Snack: Serving of fruit or vegetables in addition to drinking water.

Dinner: Fill plate with grilled, steamed, or broiled vegetable, serving of fresh fish or poultry, serving of brown rice. Drink water.

This week you'll increase your fitness activity to sixty minutes per day for five days. Again, if you have a regular routine of exercise, please continue.

Recharge your spirit through prayer and Bible study. You'll also continue your skin-care routine and get a good night's sleep. Don't forget to call and encourage your mentoring partner.

Begin Bible lesson for week three.

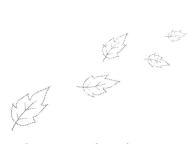

Wellness Summary Guide: Week Three

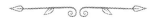

You're all phenomenal.

Wellness

Begin week three with the following steps:

1. Continue taking a vitamin supplement (optional).
2. Eat a minimum of three to four servings of fruit daily.
3. Eat a minimum of five to eight servings of different vegetables a day.
4. Drink eight glasses of water per day. Eight ounces per glass.
5. Eat one serving of protein (fresh fish or poultry) or two servings of plant protein each day. If you chose to eat meat, that's your protein. If you chose beans, that's your protein. Don't eat them together this week. Only one of them. Revisit portion size if unsure. There is no limit on your serving of vegetables, but your portion of meat protein are set each day. If you're a vegetarian, you may use other protein sources, but no dairy.
6. Eat a maximum of four times weekly one serving of complex carbohydrates.

Fitness

1. Exercise sixty minutes per day for five days.

Beauty

1. Continue a complete skin-care routine.
2. Continue to get a good night's sleep.

Spiritual

1. Recharge your spirit through prayer and Bible study.
2. Write your daily confession.

Mentoring

1. Call and encourage your mentoring partner. Reach out to a friend that you haven't talked to in a while. Let's be mindful that we all have busy lives, but we are all brothers and sisters in Christ committed one to another in this Christian walk of faith and victory.

Revive Program Notes

_____

_____

_____

_____

_____

_____

_____

_____

_____

_____

_____

_____

_____

_____

_____

_____

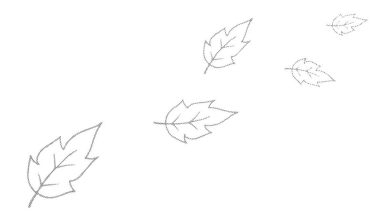

Revive Bible Lesson

Vision, Change, and Transformation

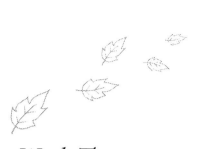

Revive Bible Lesson: Week Three

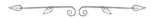

Mental Secret Number Four: Visualize success.

"And the Lord answered me, and said, write the vision, and make it plain upon tables, that he may run that readeth it. For the vision is yet for an appointed time, but at the end it shall speak, and not lie: though it tarry, wait for it; because it will surely come, it will not tarry" (Habakkuk 2:2–3).

Bible Lesson Three
Time: Fifteen minutes

Study Questions

3.1. A vision as defined in Webster's Dictionary is "the power of sight; the ability to see an image created in the imagination; a supernatural appearance." Why do you think it's necessary to have a vision in mind when you begin this program?

3.2. Read Proverbs 29: 18. Discuss its meaning as it relates to you and this program. Take the verses apart and analyze each.

3.3. Write your vision for this program. What do you see at the end of seven weeks? What do you see for the rest of your life?

3.4. Read Habakkuk 2:2–3 above. Separate each sentence. Meditate on each. How do these scriptures apply to you?

3.5. Meditate on Philippians 4:13 and Philippians 1:6. Write your thoughts.

3.6. This is week number three; have you experienced change? This can be in your mind body or spirit. Write your changes, positive or negative. Next write what you want to improve and why.

Revive Program Notes

_____

_____

_____

_____

_____

_____

_____

_____

_____

_____

_____

_____

_____

_____

_____

_____

_____

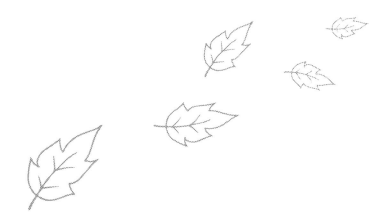

Discipline and Accountability

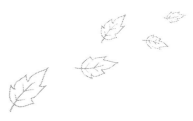

Wellness: Week Four

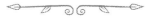

Are you singing hallelujah yet? I am. This is the halfway mark. If you've been following the program, you should be experiencing the inquisitions stage right about now. You know, questions and statements such as; What are you doing? You look different. Your skin is glowing. Are you losing weight? You seem more focused. If you're looking and feeling good, Let's give God the glory. All the praise goes to him.

I encourage you to stay committed. This is about the time in the program when our lives appear to get exceptionally busy, and everything is more important than being disciplined. Don't give up before the harvest. Stay focus on your goals and always remember, God is a rewarder of those who diligently seek him. In addition to your Revive Bible lessons, are you spending more time with God? Listen to him and learn to hear his voice. Confirm your vision and purpose and begin to work toward it.

Let's get started with week four. For your nutritional intake this week, you'll do everything that you did last week, and we will add another nutritional step. You'll begin week four by continuing to take a vitamin supplement (optional). You'll continue to eat a minimum of three to four servings of fresh fruits daily, you'll continue to eat a minimum of five to eight servings of fresh vegetables a day. Each serving should be at least one-half cup. You'll continue to drink eight glasses of water a day. (Each glass should be eight ounces). You'll continue to eat protein daily. This may be a meat serving of fresh fish or poultry each day, or if you're a vegetarian, plant foods are appropriate. Keep in mind that the meat serving size, fish or poultry, should be about the size of the palm of your hand. You'll add at least one serving of complex carbohydrates, no more than four a week.

In addition to all of the above you may add soy which is optional as the addition this week. As I continued my quest for health, I stumbled across soy and the many health benefits revealed. Soy or soy beans are fruit or seeds of a leguminous plant that has been recognized as plant food that's high in protein. It's sold in most stores, markets, wellness centers, and health food stores as a protein supplement. *The Journal of Nutrition*, Oxford Academic give soy a glowing report.

In a 2008 study, "Health Effects of Soy Protein and Isoflavones in Humans," Choa Wu Xiao explains that soy foods may contribute to lower incidents of coronary heart disease, atherosclerosis, type 2 diabetes, and decrease risk of certain types of carcinogenesis such as breast cancer and prostate cancer as well as better bone health and relief from menopausal symptoms. After discovering the numerous benefits that soy provides to our health, I added this to my diet, and it has since been incorporated into this program as an option. Check with your doctor to determine if you have any allergies to soy. If so, don't add. Just repeat week three.

Soy can be used in a variety of ways. Soy can be made into milk, it can be made into tofu which can be a meat substitute, and it can be pulverized into protein or used as a soup. Soy milk can be used in virtually anything from cereal, smoothies, cooking, or drinking. Soy beans may be purchased in most markets and health food stores in many forms. Soy beans may be purchased fresh or frozen. The beans can be roasted into nuts for snacking, or they may be boiled in the shell for about three minutes and eaten as a snack right out of the shell.

Tofu is a white block of soy cheese made from soy milk. It's sold immersed in water in sixteen- to nineteen-ounce packages. Tofu takes on the flavor of other foods and spices that it's mixed with. It's sold in three different densities, soft, firm, and extra firm. Tofu can be grilled, it can be put in vegetables, soups or made as a custard. Soy can also be purchased as tempeh, which is fermented whole soy beans that can also be used as a meat substitute. Feel free to try some of the recipes in the recipe section of your Revive book.

Let's move to fitness. This week we will continue your fitness activity for sixty minutes or one hour per day for five days, and again, if you have a regular routine, please continue.

You'll continue to recharge your spirit through prayer and Bible study and write your daily confession in your journal. Continue your skin-care routine and get a good night's sleep. Continue to build your mentor relationships and explore time to exercise together or to share the word of God.

Begin Bible lesson for week four.

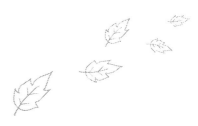

Wellness Summary Guide Week Four

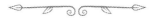

What a glorious journey. We are halfway there. I encourage you to stay committed. God is a rewarder of those who diligently seek him.

Wellness

Begin week four with the following steps:

1. Continue to taking vitamin supplements (optional).
2. Eat a minimum of three to four servings of fruit daily.
3. Eat a minimum of five to eight servings of different vegetables a day.
4. Drink eight glasses of water per day. Eight ounces per glass.
5. Eat one serving of protein (fresh fish or poultry) or two servings of plant protein each day. If you chose to eat meat that's your protein. If you chose beans, that's your protein. Don't eat them together this week. Only one of them. Revisit portion size if unsure. There is no limit on your servings of vegetables, but your portion size of meat protein is set each day. If you're a vegetarian, you may use other protein sources, but no dairy.
6. Eat a maximum of four times weekly one serving of complex carbohydrates.
7. Add soy products to your diet (optional).

Fitness

1. Exercise sixty minutes per day for five days.

Beauty

1. Continue a complete skin-care routine.
2. Continue to get a good night's sleep.

Spiritual

1. Recharge your spirit through prayer and Bible study.
2. Write your daily confession.

Mentoring

1. Continue to build your mentoring relationship. Explore times to exercise together or time to share the word of God.

Revive Program Notes

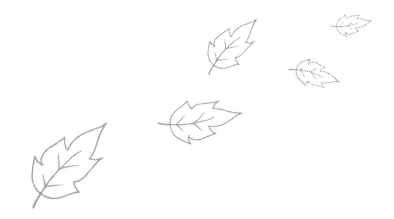

Revive Bible Lesson

Discipline and Accountability

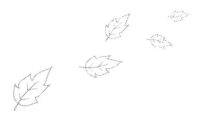

Revive Bible Lesson: Week Four

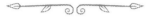

Mental Secret Number Five: Hold yourself accountable.

"And the man said, the woman whom thou gravest to be with me, she gave me of the tree, and I did eat" (Genesis 3:12).

Bible Lesson Four
Time: Fifteen minutes

Study Questions

4.1. What does accountability mean to you? Who are we ultimately accountable to? Read Romans 14:12. Complete your answers in the space provided.

4.2. Who is Adam blaming for his conduct or actions in Genesis 3:12? Why? Who should bear the blame for Adam's sin?

4.3. How can you apply accountability to this program?

4.4. Write as many words as you can think of that mean the same thing as the word *discipline.*

4.5. Read Job 36:10–11. In your own words what do you think the scripture is saying, and how can you apply it to this program?

4.6. Read Revelations 3:21. What does God promise to them that overcome?

4.7. Read Job 11:14. What does this scripture tell us to do? How can you apply the scriptures to this program?

Revive Program Notes

_____

_____

_____

_____

_____

_____

_____

_____

_____

_____

_____

_____

_____

_____

_____

_____

_____

_____

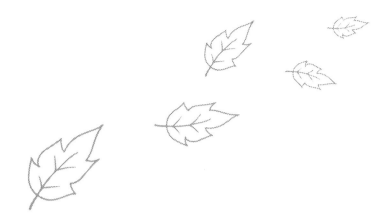

Perseverance and Encouragement

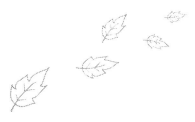

Wellness: Week Five

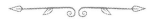

As we begin this week, it goes without saying that you're all to be truly commended for sticking to the program. May the Lord continue to let his light shine upon each of you in every area of your life.

For your nutritional intake each week, I repeat the steps because I don't want you to get lost, flip pages back and forth, or question if you've missed something. By this time, it's pretty clear that this is a lifestyle change, and you have the formula, so there's no need to continue to be repetitious, because you're doing it now as a part of your daily nutrition routine. It's fairly clear that for your nutritional intake this week you'll be doing everything that you did the last four weeks and adding another nutrition source. Simply refer to your program summary guide for the week to make sure that you're on track.

In addition to doing everything that you did last week, you'll add more fiber. What is fiber? In answering this question, I discovered that fiber is roughage. In a review of fiber published May 21, 2001, by Pacific Beach Urgent Care, "High-Fiber Diet," I read, "Fiber is the part of plant food that can't be digested by humans and it helps to keep our bowels working regularly." The review further clarifies that fiber helps to prevent constipation, and also helps to reduce the chances of getting colon cancer and heart disease, and also slows the breakdown of carbohydrates that causes a rise in blood sugar.

There are two forms of fiber: soluble fiber and insoluble fiber. The US National Library of Medicine in a 2018 review, "Soluble vs Insoluble Fiber," implies that soluble fiber may lower risk of heart disease. It also adds bulk to stool to help food pass more quickly through the stomach and intestines. It appears we need fiber to stay healthy. Although fiber is found in many sources such as fruit, bread, cereals, vegetables, nuts, legumes, and grains, some of the best sources of fiber I discovered as I continued my journey are fruits such as apples, bananas, peaches, strawberries, kiwis, and pears. So please make an effort to eat fruits and vegetables with the skin on them. For bread, this would be whole grain, bran, and seed. Bran muffins, I found, are good sources of fiber, but in some cases, depending on what is in them, they may contain high amounts of fat. So, if you're purchasing bran muffins, make sure you read the label. If you're making them from scratch, eliminate butter and maybe use olive oil or canola oil as a substitute. For legumes, in reading labels, lima beans, kidney beans, and lentils appear to be the highest sources of fiber.

For fitness this week, you'll continue your fitness activity for one hour a day for five days, and if you have an established exercise routine, please continue.

Spiritually, build up your spirit through prayer, Bible study, and praise. Try composing a victory song and sing it as often as you like.

For beauty, continue your skin-care routine and get a good night's sleep.

Mentoring, continue to build your mentoring relationship and always reevaluate your goals. Try scheduling a spa day or any activity that allows you to relax, laugh, and have fun.

Begin Bible lesson for week five.

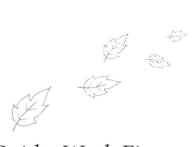

Wellness Summary Guide: Week Five

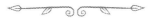

I would like to take this opportunity to commend you all for sticking with the program.

Wellness

Begin week five with the following steps:

1. Continue taking a vitamin supplement (optional).
2. Eat a minimum of three to four servings of fruit daily.
3. Eat a minimum of five to eight servings of different vegetables a day.
4. Drink eight glasses of water per day. Eight ounces per glass.
5. Eat one serving of protein (fresh fish or poultry) or two servings of plant protein each day. If you chose to eat meat, that's your protein. If you chose beans, that's your protein. Don't eat them together this week. Only eat one of them. Revisit portion size if unsure. There's no limit on your serving of vegetables, but your portion of meat proteins is set each day. If you're a vegetarian, you may use other protein sources, but no dairy.
6. Eat a maximum of four times weekly, one serving of complex carbohydrates.
7. Add soy products to your diet (optional).
8. Add more fiber to your diet.

Fitness

1. Exercise sixty minutes per day for five days.
2. Find a marathon to run or walk for a good cause.

Beauty

1. Continue a complete skin-care routine.
2. Continue to get a good night's sleep.

Spiritual

1. Build your spirit through prayer, Bible study, and song.
2. Compose your victory song and sing it as often as you like.

Mentoring

1. Continue to build your mentoring relationship.
2. Reevaluate your goals together.

Revive Program Notes

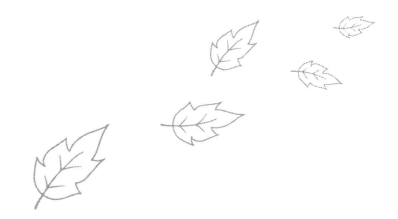

Revive Bible Lesson

Perseverance and Encouragement

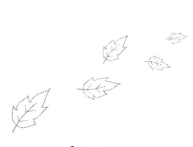

Revive Bible Lesson: Week Five

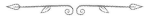

Mental Secret Number Six: Maintain a record.

"Be thou diligent to know the state of thy flocks and look well on thy herds" (Proverbs 27:23).

"Let us hold fast the profession of our faith without wavering; for he is faithful that promised" (Hebrew 10:23).

"Wherefore comfort yourselves together, and edify one another, even as also ye do" (1 Thessalonians 5:11).

Bible Lesson Five
Time: Fifteen minutes

Study Questions

5.1. Write as many words as you can think of that are used in the Bible to mean the same thing as *perseverance*.

5.2. Read Hebrews 10:23. What do you sense that God is saying to you?

5.3. Read 1 Corinthians 3:14, then ask yourself what your personal reward is for continuing this program?

5.4. Rewrite your goals and expectations for this program. Next read Mark 11:24. Rewrite this scripture, incorporating your goals into your personal prayer.

5.5. How does your relationship with your mentoring partner indicate the kind of relationship you have with God?

5.6. Read Hebrews 10:24–25. How does this apply to your mentoring relationship? Write your answer, and next reaffirm your commitment to your mentoring partner.

Revive Program Notes

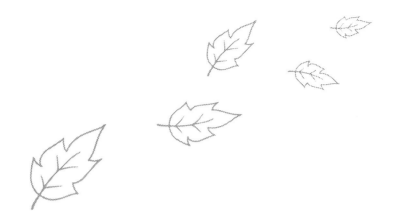

Wisdom and Knowledge

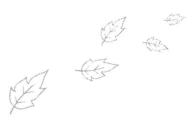

Wellness Program: Week Six

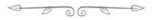

For some of you, this program has been a long time coming, but something or someone always seems to gets in the way. There have been a number of times when you've had a desire to begin this journey to being whole, but who or what was the biggest obstacle?

Let's be real. You. Own it. We all have had every excuse in the book and then some. I don't have time to exercise. I have a demanding job. I don't want to prepare separate meals, because my family will not eat healthy. I just don't want to give up my treats. And on and on, we go. Well, look at yourself now and say, "The pity party is over. I'm on the move, and there's nothing that can stop me now." If you've faithfully followed the program, hug yourself and take a bow. You earned it. Running the race and being able to see the finish line is phenomenal. You're now in week six. You're too close to the finish line. Don't slow down and lose focus. Keep going.

For your nutritional intake this week, again you'll do everything that you did for the last five weeks, but you'll add another nutritional step. You'll add necessary or essential fats to your diet. Adding necessary or essential fats to your diet is a good thing. However, before I embark on why they're a good thing, I'll give you a brief overview of fats or fatty acids.

Fatty acids are classified as saturated and unsaturated fats. In *Prescription for Nutritional Healing: The A-to-Z Guide to Supplements*, Phyllis A. Balch, CNC, points out that saturated fats can significantly raise the blood cholesterol level, especially the (LDS) or bad cholesterol. In *The Longevity Prescription: The 8 Proven Keys to a Long, Healthy*

Life, Robert N. Butler, MD, emphasizes that saturates fats should be limited because these fats tend to elevate blood cholesterol levels, putting you at greater risk for strokes and heart attacks. The American Heart Association in a March 2017 review of saturated fats recommended that we limit saturated fats, which are found in butter, cheese, red meat, and other animal-based foods.

Unsaturated fats, according to Brenda Watson, CNC, and Leonard Smith, MD, in the *Fiber35 Diet: Nature's Weight Loss Secrets*, are the good fats that we should include in our diets every day. Necessary or essential fats are also classes of unsaturated fats. These fatty acids, I learned, are fatty oils or fatty acids that the body needs for good health. They are essential because we need them to live.

Most medical guides including *The American Medical Association Family Medical Guide* lists the two basic categories of essential fatty acids as omega-3 and omega-6. These essential fats, according to the 2016 Nutrition and Health Information Guide published by the Center for Nutrition in Schools, Department of Nutrition, University of California Davis, are ones that our bodies are unable to make and that we need to obtain from food.

Authors Eric J. Chan, MD, and Leslie Cho, MD, in a study called "What Can We Expect from Omega-3 Fatty Acids?" published by The Cleveland Clinic Journal of Medicine, also reinforces the fact that omega-3 is essential, is found in plant sources, can't be manufactured by the body, and must be obtained from our diets. In essence, we must rely on the foods we ingest to get them into our bodies.

Phyllis A. Balch, CNC, in *Prescription for Nutritional Healing: The A-to-Z Guide to Supplements*, indicates that these essential fatty acids have a desirable effect on many disorders. They improve skin and hair, reduce blood cholesterol, reduce blood-clot formation, and are essential for rebuilding and producing new cells. Omega-3 fatty acids, according to *The American Medical Association Family Medical Guide*, help to protect the heart, improve cholesterol levels, and reduce joint pain and inflammation, and are found in fatty fish such as mackerel and salmon. They're also found in deep-green vegetables.

Another source of omega-3 fatty acids are flax seed and flax seed oil. Nina Shandler in *Estrogen: The Natural Way* identifies flax seed as the potentially richest source of plant estrogen. In addition to being high in omega-3 fatty acids, flax seed is also a good source for fiber as indicated in the *Complete Food & Nutrition Guide.*

The other fatty acid is omega-6. Most omega-6 fatty acids come from green vegetables, nuts, seeds, avocados, grains, and cooking oils. So, this week, I want you, to add more omega-3 and omega-6 fatty acids to your diet. Some of the omega-3 and omega-6 fatty acids have already been included in the form of green, leafy vegetables and fish, but as another source of omega-3 fatty acid, add flax seed to your diet. You can find flax seed in most health food stores and some major super markets. Flax seed can also be found in cereal, bread and crackers. Make it a habit to read the labels carefully for all ingredients. Flax seed can be used to make muffins, it can be sprinkled on salads, or you can simply add a teaspoon to your smoothies in the morning. As you begin to read labels, you'll find that flax seed is also a good source of fiber.

This week, you'll continue your fitness activity for one hour a day, or you may increase if time permits. Recharge your spirit through prayer and Bible study. Continue your comprehensive skin-care routine and get a good night's sleep. Continue to build your mentoring relationships.

Begin week-six Bible lesson.

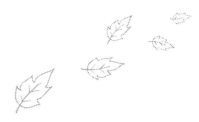

Wellness Summary Guide: Week Six

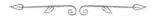

"Know ye not that they which run in a race run all, but one receiveth the prize? So, run that ye may obtain" (1 Corinthians 9:24).

Wellness

Begin week six with the following steps:

1. Continue taking vitamin supplements (optional).
2. Eat a minimum of three to four servings of fruit daily.
3. Eat a minimum of five to eight servings of different vegetables a day.
4. Drink eight glasses of water per day. Eight ounces per glass.
5. Eat one serving of protein (fresh fish or poultry) or two servings of plant protein each day. If you chose to eat meat, that's your protein. If you chose beans, that's your protein. Don't eat them together this week. Only one of them. Revisit portion size if unsure. There's no limit on your servings of vegetables, but your portion size of meat protein is set each day. If you're a vegetarian, you may use other protein sources, but no dairy.
6. Eat a maximum of four times weekly one serving of complex carbohydrates.
7. Add soy products to your diet (optional).
8. Add more fiber to your diet.
9. Add necessary or essential fats to your diet.

Fitness

1. In addition to exercising sixty minutes a day, try adding a dance or yoga class for fun and relaxation.

Beauty

1. Continue a complete skin-care routine.
2. Continue to get a good night's sleep.

Spiritual

1. Build your spirit through prayer, Bible study, and song.
2. Compose your victory song and sing it as often as you like.
3. Reach out to a friend and pray with them.

Mentoring

1. Continue to build your mentoring relationship.
2. Speak words of encouragement.
3. Write your daily confession and share with your mentoring partner.

Revive Program Notes

_____

_____

_____

_____

_____

_____

_____

_____

_____

_____

_____

_____

_____

_____

_____

_____

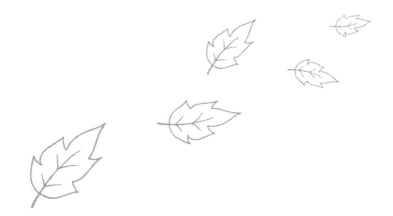

Revive Bible Lesson

Wisdom and Knowledge

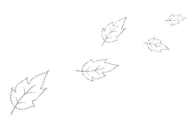

Revive Bible Lesson: Week Six

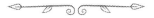

Mental Secret Number Seven: Rebound and learn from your mistakes.

"Grace and peace be multiplied unto you through the knowledge of God, and of Jesus our Lord. According as his divine power hath given unto us all things that pertains unto life and godliness, through the knowledge of him that hath called us to glory and virtue. For if these things be in you, and abound, they make you that ye shall neither be barren nor unfruitful in the knowledge of our Lord Jesus Christ. But he that lacketh these things is blind, and cannot see afar off, and hath forgotten that he was purged from his old sins" (2 Peter 1:2–3, 8–9).

Bible Study Lesson Six
Time: Fifteen minutes

Study Questions

6.1. Read Proverbs 4:7, 22. How does God's word define wisdom? What does God's word say wisdom is to us? Underline the words, circle them, and engrave them in your memory. Next write your thoughts.

6.2. Read Proverb 4:10–11, 13 and John 8:32. What does God want you to learn, understand, and practice from these scriptures?

6.3. Read James 4:7. This program is personal to you. Write your personal confession to God, then reaffirm your commitment to this program.

6.4. Read Colossian 2:21. Reword the scripture into your personal prayer.

6.5. Read James 1:22, 25. What does these scriptures tell you if you continue to be a doer of God's word?

Revive Program Notes

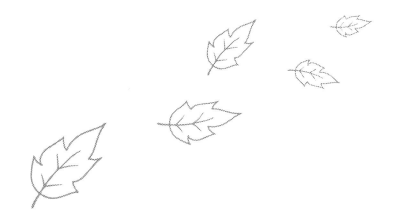

Victory and Revelation

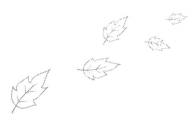

Wellness: Week Seven

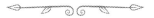

You're now in the final week of the program. Could you have made it through without Jesus? You're victorious. You're more than a conqueror. You're truly an overcomer. As you begin the last and final week of the program, just know that this does not end your journey. This is a lifestyle change for you to be continued. Think about how far you've come—not just with your health but with your spiritual walk, your relationships with others, and any other areas in your life that you see change. Take a moment and thank God for your victory.

At the end of this week, you'll take a picture, weigh yourself, and remeasure yourself just as you did at the beginning of the program. You'll record your answers in your Revive book in week one on the same page as before. Then you'll compare the difference. If you participated in the program as a group, when you meet again, you'll give your testimony.

For your nutritional intake this week, you'll do everything that you've done in the past six weeks. You'll also add an additional step. Yes, just one more step. This week, you'll be adding more variety to your diet. You'll add a variety of new and different food sources that are rich in protein and niacin. These foods are not required but may be used as a substitute to break the boredom of eating the same things weekly. If you have allergies to gluten, don't add these to your diet. However, you may find these in the gluten-free section in some health food stores.

The first new grain is quinoa. In reading labels, I discovered that it's rich in protein and can be used as a substitute for potatoes and rice. This is also sold in most supermarkets and health food stores. The second new grain is couscous. This can be used as a substitute for pasta or rice. Food labels indicate that it's rich in protein and high in fiber. Couscous comes in regular wheat or whole wheat. Whole-wheat couscous if you have no allergies is the one to incorporate into your nutrition plan. The third addition is wild rice. Again, in reading labels, it appears to be high in proteins and a good source of fiber.

As with the past weeks, you'll continue your fitness activities. Continue to build your spirit through prayer and Bible study and give God praises. Continue your complete skin-care routine and get a good night's sleep. Take the time to congratulate your mentoring partner and support team on a job well done.

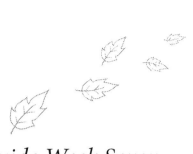

Wellness Summary Guide Week Seven

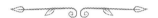

"Oh, what a friend we have in Jesus, for we are victorious. We are more than conquers. We are overcomers."

Wellness

Begin week seven with the following steps:

1. Continue taking vitamin supplements (optional).
2. Eat a minimum of three to four servings of fruit daily.
3. Eat a minimum of five to eight servings of different vegetables a day.
4. Drink eight glasses of water per day. Eight ounces per glass.
5. Eat one serving of protein (fresh fish or poultry) or two servings of plant protein each day. If you chose to eat meat, that's your protein. If you chose beans, that's your protein. Don't eat them together this week. Only one of them. Revisit portion size if unsure. There's no limit on your servings of vegetables, but your portion size of meat protein is set each day. If you're a vegetarian, you may use other protein sources, but no dairy.
6. Eat a maximum of four times weekly one serving of complex carbohydrates.
7. Add soy products to your diet (optional).
8. Add more fiber to your diet.
9. Add necessary or essential fats to your diet.
10. Add more variety to your diet.

Fitness

1. In addition to exercising sixty minutes a day, think about and prepare to broaden your horizons. Run a marathon in the near future.

Beauty

1. Continue a complete skin-care routine.
2. Continue to get a good night's sleep.

Spiritual

1. Build your spirit through prayer, Bible study, and song.
2. Compose your victory song and sing it as often as you like.
3. Reaching out and pray with a friend.

Mentoring

1. Congratulate your mentoring partner on a job well done.
2. Record your progress.

Revive Program Notes

_____

_____

_____

_____

_____

_____

_____

_____

_____

_____

_____

_____

_____

_____

_____

_____

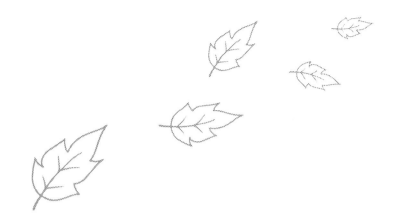

Revive Bible Lesson

Victory and Revelation

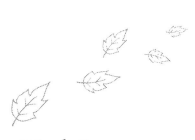

Revive Bible Lesson: Week Seven

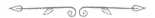

"His Lord said unto him, "Well done, thou good and faithful servant; you have been faithful over a few things; I will make thee ruler over many things; enter thou into the joy of thy Lord" (Matthew 25:21).

Bible Lesson Seven
Time: Fifteen minutes

Study Questions

7.1. Why do you believe God led you to go through this program? Pray and meditate on this question, then write your answer. Read Proverbs 3:1–6.

7.2. Read Isaiah 40:5 and Philippians 2:13. Revisit question number one and review your answer.

7.3. Read John 16:13 and 1 Corinthians 2:9–10. Reflect on these scriptures in your private moments.

7.4. Only the spirit of God knows what God is doing in your life. Ask him what he wants you to do as a result of going through this program? Pray and wait on his answer.

Revive Program Notes

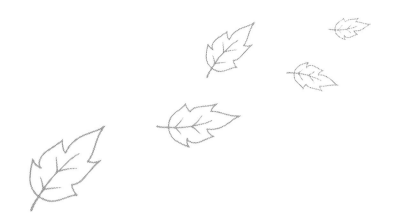

Revive Recipes

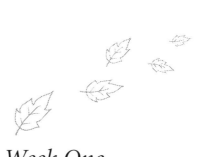

Revive Recipes: Week One

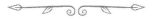

Fasting and cleansing

Smoothies

Early Bird
2 stalks of celery
1 apple
1 orange
1/2 lemon
1 carrot
Fresh ginger to taste
Add water as needed
Wash and cut all fruits and vegetables to fit in blender or food processor. Process foods for about fifteen seconds, pour in glass, and drink immediately. Refrigerate all unused portions.

Heavenly Smoothie
1 peeled banana
1/2 cup of strawberries
1/2 cup of peaches
1 cup of water
Wash and cut all fruit in medium to small pieces. Place all fruit in blender or food processor. Blend for about fifteen seconds or until smooth, adding more water if needed. Pour in glass and drink. For best results, try freezing fruit prior to use. You may use any combination of

your favorite fruits to make a smoothie. (In week four, you may use soy or almond milk.)

Green Drink
1/2 cup fresh spinach
1/2 cup of fresh kale
1/2 cup of fresh dandelions
1/2 fresh orange
1/2 banana
Hint of fresh ginger
1/2 cup of cranberries fresh or frozen
1/2 mango (optional)
1 1/2 cups of water
Place all ingredients in food processor or blender. Process for about fifteen seconds or until smooth. Add more water if needed. Pour into glass and drink. For best results, try freezing fruit prior to use. You may use any combination of your favorite fruits to make a smoothie.

Fruit Medley
You may cut up any combination of your favorite fresh fruits in a bowl to make a medley.
Always wash all fruit thoroughly prior to use.

Salads
Use any combination of greens and your favorite vegetables to make your salads. Add your favorite dressing to taste. (Don't add corn.)

Quick Cucumber Salad
1 large tomato chopped in bite size pieces
1 large cucumber peeled and chopped into bite size pieces
1 garlic clove minced
4 tablespoons of rice vinegar
2 teaspoon olive oil
Salt and pepper to taste (optional)
You may add fresh dill for variety.

Place all ingredients in medium-size bowl, toss until cucumber, tomatoes, and garlic are completely coated. Cover and place in refrigerator until ready to serve.

Vegetables Rolls
8 to 10 whole red, green, or butter lettuce leaves.
1 medium carrot grated
1/2 red or yellow pepper sliced thin
1/2 green pepper sliced thin
1/2 cucumber sliced thin
1/2 cup bean sprouts
1 small can of sliced olives drained
1 small tomato sliced thin
1 quarter red onion sliced thin
Wash and clean all vegetables prior to use. Pat lettuce dry with paper towels. On a clean surface, place one whole lettuce leaf flat. For best results, add in this order. In mid-center of lettuce leaf, lay cucumber slices, tomato slices, carrots, peppers, bean sprouts, and olives. Fold short side of leaf over vegetables and roll, tucking ends as you roll. Secure with a toothpick if needed. Dip in your favorite dressing. Place all uneaten rolls in refrigerator in a sealed container. You may add apple slices for variety.

Marinated or Sauté Vegetable Medley
1 cup of asparagus chopped into quarters
1 cup brussels sprouts cut in halves
1 cup of carrots sliced diagonally
1 cup of broccoli crowns
1/4 cup of green onions chopped
2 garlic cloves crushed
3/4 cup of rice vinegar
1/2 cup of olive oil
1/2 cup of red radishes sliced (optional for salad)
1 cup each of yellow and red peppers sliced thin
1 cup of cauliflower

Wisk rice vinegar and oil together in a separate bowl. Combine vegetables in large plastic bag. Add oil and vinegar mixture, sealed and shake gently making sure all vegetables are coated. Let marinate for one hour. Shake gently prior to serving. Pour in a large bowl and enjoy. For sauté vegetables, see recipe below.

Steamed Vegetables
Use any combination of your favorite fresh vegetables, add salt and pepper to taste or your favorite spice or seasonings. Place in steamer for about three minutes. Steam longer for softer vegetables. Don't use any butter, oil, margarine, cheese, or sauces.

Sauté Vegetables
Simply heat three tablespoons of olive oil in large sauté pan or wok, add all vegetables, turning gently for about three minutes. You may cook longer for softer vegetables.

Vegetable Soup
1 small green cabbage shredded.
1/2 small onion chopped
2 garlic cloves chopped
1 large carrots chopped or sliced diagonally
1 cup broccoli crowns
1 can chopped tomatoes, 20 ounces
1 small yellow squash cubed
1 small zucchini squash cubed (optional)
1/2 green pepper chopped
1/2 red pepper chopped
3 to 4 cups of vegetable stock as needed
2 tablespoon of olive oil
Salt and pepper to taste
Clean all vegetables prior to use. In large pot, heat two tablespoons of olive oil, sauté onions and garlic for one minute. Add vegetable stock and bring to a boil. Add all other ingredients and reduce heat. Cook for five minutes for crunchy vegetables. Cook longer for softer vegetables.

Let stand for five minutes before serving. In week two, you may use chicken broth as a substitute.

Fresh Asparagus
1 bunch of fresh asparagus
2 tablespoon of soy sauce
1 tablespoon of olive oil
Garlic powder to taste or fresh garlic chopped finely
Salt and pepper to taste
Cut tough ends off of asparagus. Using a peeler remove fibrous outer layer. Place asparagus on cookie sheet, sprinkle all other ingredients over asparagus, turning until evenly coated. Place in oven on broil for about three to five minutes. Turn once to cook each side. Remove from oven and serve.

Desserts
1 banana peeled and sliced diagonally
1/2 mango
1/2 cup of strawberries or any berries of your choice. May use frozen berries if fresh is not available.
Chill banana in freezer for about five minutes. Puree berries and mango in food processor, take banana from freezer, pour puree on top, and enjoy. You may use any fruit of your choice for a toping.

Revive Recipes: Week Two

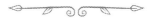

Protein

Grilled Portobello Mushrooms
4 large portobello mushrooms
2 garlic cloves crushed
1/2 cup of water
1 tablespoon of olive oil
1/2 teaspoon of fresh ginger
2 tablespoons of honey
3 tablespoons of soy sauce
Clean mushrooms, removing stem from center, and place in large glass dish. In a medium bowl, add crushed garlic, ginger, soy sauce, olive oil, honey, and water. Mix well, pour over mushrooms, cover with plastic wrap, and place in refrigerator to marinate for thirty minutes, turning on both sides occasionally. Spray grill with nonstick spray. Place mushrooms on grill and cook for five minutes or until mushrooms are tender. Remove from grill and serve.

Stuffed Tomatoes
3 large tomatoes cut in half
2 cooked chicken breasts cubed
1 stalk of celery
1/2 cup of green onions
1 medium carrots
1/2 cup of red cabbage
2 garlic cloves

1/2 cup of parsley
Dressing of choice to taste
Salt and pepper to taste
Wash all vegetables. Remove or scoop out insides of tomatoes. Place tomatoes on a serving platter. In food processor, add celery, onions, carrots, garlic, and cabbage. Process until all ingredients are finely chopped. Place in a large bowl. Cut chicken breast into chunks place in food process for about five seconds. Pour in bowl with other ingredients; add dressing of choice and mix well. Scoop into hollow tomatoes, garnish with parsley, and serve. You can use tuna as a substitute for chicken.

Grilled Salmon or Chicken
4 6-ounce salmon fillets
Garlic powder to taste
Salt and pepper to taste
Olive oil spray
Seasoned salmon with garlic powder, salt, and pepper. Cover with plastic wrap and place in refrigerator for about twenty minutes. Preheat broiler or grill. Brush salmon on both sides with olive oil. Place salmon on grill and grill for about three minutes on each side or until fish is flakey. Place on serving platter with your favorite vegetable.

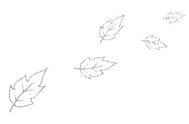

Revive Recipes: Week Three

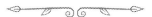

Complex Carbohydrates

Breakfast
Whole-grain oatmeal

Quick Rice Medley
1 1/2 cups brown rice cooked
1/2 cup of frozen green peas rinsed
1/2 cup of carrots grated
1/2 cup red peppers chopped or sliced
1/2 cup of green onions chopped
2 garlic cloves crushed
2 tablespoon of olive oil
1/2 cup of vegetable or chicken broth
Salt and pepper to taste
Cook rice in your usual manner. Place cooked rice in large mixing bowl. In microwave dish, mix broth, peas, olive oil, carrots, red peppers onion, and garlic. Cover and place in microwave for about two minutes or until vegetables are tender. Remove and add to rice. Mix well. Add salt and pepper to taste. Serve with your favorite protein and vegetables.

Salad in a Sandwich
3 pieces of whole-wheat pita bread
8 to 10 leaves of red, green, or butter leaf lettuce. (You may also use romaine lettuce.)
1 medium tomato sliced thin

1 medium-size cucumber sliced thin
1 cup of sprouts
1/2 red pepper sliced thin
1/2 green pepper sliced thin
1/2 yellow pepper sliced thin
1/2 cup of red cabbage shredded
1 avocado sliced in strips
1 large carrot grated
Salad dressing of choice

Cut each piece of pita bread in half. Open bread in center (cut side up) and place all ingredients inside. Layer as follows: Add lettuce, tomato, cucumbers and avocado on one side of bread. Mix all other ingredients in a separate bowl with your favorite dressing. Scoop equal amounts into pita pockets and enjoy.

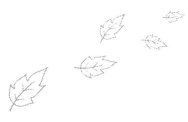

Revive Recipes: Week Four

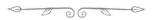

Soy

Cereals
Whole-grain, multigrain, wheat, or soy. Check with your doctor to make sure that you don't have allergies.

Green Beans and Tofu
8 oz. of firm or extra-firm tofu
4 teaspoons of honey
3 cups of fresh or frozen cut green beans
4 tablespoon of olive oil
1 teaspoon of sesame seed oil
2 garlic cloves crushed
1/2 teaspoon of fresh ginger finely grated
6 tablespoons of soy sauce
2 cups of water
Nonstick canola or olive oil spray
In medium-size bowl, add three teaspoons of soy sauce, one garlic clove crushed, two teaspoons olive oil, two teaspoon honey, and water. Mix well. Remove tofu from water and cut into cubes. Place in bowl with prepared liquid. Toss until all pieces are coated. Let tofu marinate for about thirty minutes. Remove the tofu from marinade. Spray frying pan or grill with nonstick spray. Grill or cook until the tofu is lightly brown on all sides. Remove from heat and set aside. Steam green beans for about two minutes in microwave and set aside. In a heavy saucepan over medium heat, add remaining olive oil, sesame oil, and garlic sauté

for about three seconds. Stir in ginger, soy sauce and honey, cook for about one minute more. Add tofu, tossing lightly. Add green beans, toss lightly to coat, remove from heat, and serve.

Tomato Tofu and Cucumber salad
1 large cucumber cubed
1 cup cherry tomatoes
1 garlic cloves minced
1 16-ounce pack of extra-firm tofu cubed
1/2 teaspoon of dill chopped fine optional
1/4 cup green onions chopped
1/2 cup of rice vinegar
2 tablespoon of olive oil
Salt and pepper to taste
Place cucumber and tomato in a medium bowl. Drain water from tofu. Cut into cubes, grill on all sides until lightly brown. Place in separate bowl. In a small bowl, add garlic, green onions, dill, olive oil, and vinegar. Wisk well and pour over cucumbers and tomatoes. Add tofu, salt, and pepper to taste. Toss lightly to coat. For a chilled salad, place in refrigerator for about ten minutes. Enjoy as a side dish.

Turkey and Soy Meatloaf
1 pound of ground turkey
1/2 package of onion soup mix
1 block of 8-ounce soft or silken tofu
1 egg
1/4 cup of onions, any kind
1/4 cup of green or red pepper
1 celery stalk
1/2 cup seasoned breadcrumbs
1 garlic clove (optional)
2 tablespoons of soy sauce
1/2 teaspoon of salt
1/2 teaspoons black pepper

In large mixing bowl, add ground turkey. In food processor, add onions, green pepper, celery, and garlic blends until finely chopped. Add to ground turkey. Place tofu in food processor with onion soup mix, blend until a smooth paste. Add to ground turkey along with bread crumbs, egg, soy sauce, salt, and black pepper. Mix well. Spray loaf pan with nonstick canola or olive oil. Place in loaf pan and bake for about forty-five to sixty minutes or until done at 350 degrees. Use your judgment if you feel it should cook longer. Remove from oven. Let stand for twenty minutes before serving.

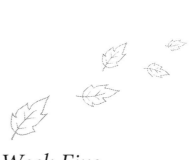

Revive Recipes: Week Five

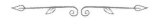

Fiber

Breakfast
1 serving of oatmeal or high-fiber breakfast cereal with soy milk

Quick Three-Bean Salad
1 cup of red kidney beans cooked
1 cup of black beans cooked
1 cup of cut green beans cooked
2 garlic cloves minced
1/4 cup of sliced red onions
1/2 cup of Italian dressing
If using canned beans. Rinse and drain liquid. Combine all ingredients in salad bowl. Mix well. Place in refrigerator and chill for twenty minutes prior to serving.

Marinated Vegetable Medley
1 cup of asparagus cut into quarters
1 cup brussels sprouts cut in halves
1 cup of carrots sliced diagonally
1 cup of cut broccoli crowns
1/4 cup of green onions chopped
2 garlic cloves crushed
1/2 cup of red radishes sliced
1/2 cup of cauliflower
1 cup of rice vinegar

1/4 cup of olive oil

½ cup each of red and yellow peppers sliced thin

Wisk rice vinegar and olive oil together in a separate bowl. Combine all other vegetables in a large plastic bag. Add oil and vinegar mixture and seal. Shake gently making sure all vegetables are coated. Let marinate for one hour. Shake gently prior to serving. Pour vegetables in large bowl and enjoy.

Navy Bean Soup

1 pound of dry navy beans

2 bay leaves

1 large carrot chopped

1/2 medium onion chopped

1 celery stalk chopped

1 8-ounce can of tomatoes chopped

2 garlic cloves chopped

1/4 cup of olive oil

3 cups chicken broth

2 cups of water

2 whole cloves

Salt and pepper to taste

Rinse the beans well, place in a large pot or bowl that allows room for the beans to expand. Cover with water and allow beans to soak for about three hours. Rinse and drain beans. Place in a large stockpot, cover with chicken broth or water, and add all other ingredients. Let cook slowly until beans are tender. Add water or chicken broth as needed. You may substitute, kidney beans, black beans, or pinto beans.

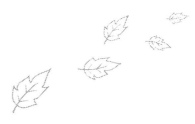

Revive Recipes: Week Six

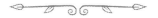

Adding Essential Fat

Breakfast
1 serving of flax cereal with almond or soy milk

Green Drink
1/2 cup fresh spinach
1/2 cup of fresh kale
1/2 cup of fresh dandelions
1/2 fresh orange
1/2 banana
Hint of fresh ginger
1/2 cup of cranberries fresh or frozen
1 teaspoon of flax seed
1 cup of water
Place all ingredients in food processor or blender. Process for about three to four seconds or until smooth. Pour into glass and drink. For best results try freezing fruit prior to use. You may use any combination of your favorite fruits to make a smoothie.

Grilled Salmon
4–6 ounces salmon fillets
Garlic powder to taste
Salt and pepper to taste
Olive oil spray

Seasoned salmon with garlic powder, salt, and pepper. Cover with plastic wrap and place in refrigerator for about twenty minutes. Preheat broiler or grill. Brush salmon on both sides with olive oil. Place salmon on grill for about three minutes on both sides until fish is flakey. Place on serving platter with your favorite vegetable.

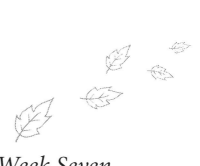

Revive Recipes: Week Seven

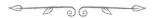

Variety

There are a number of other grains that provide variety to meal plans that are high in nutrients, such as quinoa, couscous and wild rice.

Vegetable Couscous Salad
1 1/2 cups of vegetable or chicken stock
2 cups of couscous
1/4 cup of grated carrots shredded
1/4 cup frozen green peas rinsed and thawed
2 tablespoons olive oil
2 scallions chopped
2 garlic cloves crushed
3 tablespoons cilantro chopped
Salt and pepper to taste
In sauce pan, heat oil and add scallions, garlic, and carrots. Sauté for about one minute. Add chicken or vegetable stock. Bring to a boil. Stir in couscous and green peas, salt, and pepper. Cover and remove the pan from heat. Let stand for about fifteen minutes or until couscous has swelled and all liquid is absorbed.

Quinoa Salad
2 cups of quinoa
2 cups chicken broth or water
1 cup carrots chopped
1/2 small red bell pepper chopped

1 medium cucumber seeded and chopped
1/4 cup red onion chopped
3/4 cup chopped parsley
1 large garlic clove minced
1/4 cup rice vinegar
1/4 cup lemon juice
1 tablespoon olive oil
1/2 teaspoon salt
1/2 teaspoon black pepper

Place quinoa in a fine strainer and hold under cold running water until water runs clear. Drain well. Combine water or broth in medium sauce pan with quinoa. Bring to a boil. Cover, reduce heat, and simmer until grains are translucent. Cook about fifteen minutes. Remove from heat and let it cool. Use fork to fluff lightly. In a large bowl, combine carrots, cucumber, bell pepper, onions, and parsley, and set aside. In a small bowl, combine olive oil, lemon juice, garlic, rice vinegar or red wine vinegar, salt, and pepper. Blend completely and set aside. Test quinoa to make sure it's cool and fluffed. Add to large bowl with chopped vegetables. Add dressing and mix thoroughly. Add salt and pepper to taste. Let stand for fifteen minutes before serving.

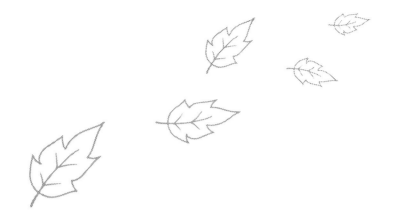

Revive Bible Study Discussions

Week One through Seven

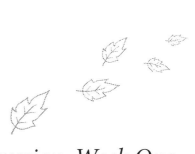

Revive Bible Study Discussion: Week One

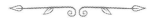

This is week one of the Revive seven-week Bible study. Don't review this segment until you've completed your personal week one Revive Bible lesson.

The Bible study begins with fasting and cleansing and centers around Mental Secret Number One: "Believe that you can do it." Our premier scripture is Mark 9:23. "Jesus said unto him, if thou canst believe, all things are possible to him that believeth." As you begin this Bible study, you'll find that this basic mental principle embodies the catalyst for change. As you strengthen your faith in God this next seven weeks and your belief in your ability to make lifestyle changes in nutrition and exercise, you'll be amazed at how this simple concept can and will affect other areas of your life,

Questions and Discussion

1.1. What does fasting mean to you?

In the past as a program facilitator, I often emphasized that this Bible study is personal. It's not a quiz, and there are no wrong answers. If you're in a group, your responses may be in an open discussion. If you have answers such as "to abstain from food" or "eat sparingly," that's great. Additional responses not listed may be "self-denial of food," "self-discipline," or "self-control." Whatever the answer, clearly, it's a sacrifice.

1.2. What does Isaiah 58:6–8 tell us about fasting? Explain its meaning and how it relates to your definition of fasting.

Fasting is voluntary. It isn't something that any of us are legally bound to do. It's a personal sacrifice of free will and a time of repentance. As I view the scriptures, fasting was used as a means of atonement or conciliation for sin. To be free from sin, you must have an earnest, heartfelt, and sincere desire to be delivered from sin. This requires a conscious recognition of temptation and the desires of the flesh. It commands a change in our attitudes or states of mind.

Food has become for some of us a bondage. When we fast, we break the yoke that's binding, then we have the victory to let go and be free. How do you personally feel after completing this first week? In your spirit? In your body? Do you feel a sense of accomplishment?

1.3. Why do you think it's necessary to cleanse your body to begin this program? After writing your answer, read Colossians 3:9–10 and Romans 6:6. Meditate on 1 Corinthians 3:16–17.

In Colossians, it appears that Paul seems to be encouraging believers to put off the old man and put on the new man by living good and virtuous lives before God. As we apply the scriptures to this program, this means to stop old habits or behaviors that you continue to engage in. As you read the scripture, the old man means to do away with old sin. The old sin as it applies to this program are your old eating habits, for example fried chicken, pizza, fried pork, excessive salt, rich and creamy foods high in fats and cholesterols.

The apostle Paul also said to put on the new man, which is learning to live righteous before God. If you're questioning how this can be done, the answer is simple. This can be done by developing healthy eating habits that produce a lifestyle change. This lifestyle change breaks the bonds of addiction to foods that cause destruction and deterioration to our bodies.

As you meditate on the assigned scripture, in Romans 6:6, be mindful that it addresses the crucifying of the body, the old man, and being free of sin. As the scripture relates to this program, it encourages us to be dead of sin and alive in Christ. When you decide to change your eating habits, you crucify the old man. You're no longer eating those things that contribute to chronic illness and ill health. When you began a lifestyle change, you crucify the old man (the old sin), and thus, it's dead.

The scripture in 1 Corinthians 3:16 says, "We are the temples of God, and the spirit of God dwells within us." Since we are God's temples, our bodies must be kept holy and set apart for the service of God and must command absolute adoration and reverence to God. Making conscious decisions to stop eating foods that contribute to ill health, and applying daily sound principals of nutrition and fitness sets our bodies apart for the service of God. When we put foods into our bodies that cause disease, strokes and heart attacks, we defile God's temple. "If any man defiles the temple of God, him shall God destroy it. For the temple of God is holy, which temple are ye?" (1 Corinthians 3:17).

1.4. Why is it necessary to have the right mind-set to begin this program? Read Proverbs 23:7. What does this mean to you?

Your frame of mind influences your personal feelings, thoughts, or attitudes, so whatever your answer is to this question, it's your sincere thought, but know that this sets the tone as you move forward in any endeavor.

The second part of this question asks you to read Proverbs 23:7. "For as he thinketh in his heart, so is he." What we feel or think about something becomes our focal point and often becomes more important than the issue at hand because, our thoughts are powerful. How we think or feel about something can and will form our attitudes toward it in our present minds. Our present minds are where we harbor our daily functions or activities. These are our joys, pains, worries, or limitations. Our present minds are those part of us that are all that we desire and hope to be.

The beauty in this is that this part is absolutely and completely under our control at all times. Just knowing this lets us know that we have the power to sort through, and choose what to throw out, or choose what should not be there.

The Bible says, "Choose this day whom you will serve" (Joshua 24:15). You are the masters of your fate. You decide whom you'll serve.

The decision is always yours, and it can't be relinquished or passed on to others. Will your mind be an open vessel for God, or will it be an open vessel for that which is unlike God?

1.5. How does Mark 9:23 apply to you in relations to this program?

"Jesus said unto him, if thou can believe, all things are possible to him that believeth." Your beliefs are your personal and sincere thoughts, and it's these thoughts that influence our actions. Most of us often express negative thoughts regarding our time. If we were to frame the title for a hit song, it would be "I Don't Have Time"—time to eat properly, time to prepare healthy food, time to exercise, time to drink water, time to take vitamins, and on and on. These are all of the things that contribute to a healthier you.

It appears that in spite of your time crises, you do have time to build bad health and contribute to and speed up your demise. Maybe, just maybe, these excuses are the results of how we think and how we prioritize. If you feel that your health is something that should be put on a back burner until such time that it can be worked into your busy schedule, then somewhere in your subconscious mind you believe that time waits for you. "For as he thinketh in his heart, so is he" (Proverbs 23:7). In essence, what you think is who you are.

Our thoughts influence our beliefs; our beliefs are that which we hold to be truths. Our beliefs dictate and often trigger our behaviors. This, in many cases, works to our good, but in some cases, it may work to our demise. So, if we believe something that becomes the catalyst of our conduct. To believe is to have the conscious state of mind of acceptance without evidence or proof. Whatever you believe, you can achieve. Keep working and moving toward your goals. You as a participant have proven this to yourself by completing this first week. It was your belief and actions that compelled you this far.

1.6. Read and meditate on Philippians 4:13 and 2 Samuels 22:33.

Continue to meditate on these scriptures as you continue the program. Memorize and recite them daily.

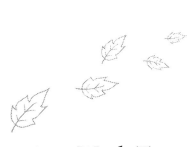

Revive Bible Study Discussion: Week Two

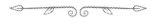

Welcome to week two of the seven-week series of the Revive Bible study. Don't review this segment until you've completed your personal week-two Revive Bible lesson.

Week-two Bible study begins with commitment and time management. It's also centered around Mental Secret Number Two: "Make an unyielding commitment," and Mental Secret Number Three: "Set realistic goals." Our premier scriptures are Romans 12:1, Proverbs 16:3, and Luke 14:28–30.

Questions and Discussion

2.1. In your own words write, what you think it means to make a commitment.

As you examine your thoughts, go beyond the surface. Dig deeper. If you have answers such as "a commitment means an agreement," "a pledge," "an obligation or a duty to something," or "a duty to someone," that's great. If you have something additional, that's wonderful also. You are now beginning your unique journey with your heavenly father. When we make commitments, we take a vow of trust to stand firm and honor our words and actions now and in the future.

2.2. What choices have you made concerning your commitment to Jesus?

This is your personal commitment as this Bible study is personal to you. "Thou shall love the Lord thy God with all thy heart, and with all thy soul and with all thy mind. This is the first and greatest commandment" (Matthew 22:37–38). The apostle Paul was a flawless model of commitment to Jesus. I was fortunate some years ago to hear Dr. Charles Stanley minister on commitment, and it left a lasting impression. He implied that when you make a commitment to Jesus, you're all in, not halfway. The apostle Paul was devoted to serving God throughout all of the times he was imprisoned for simply doing what God called him to do. He did not allow his circumstances to deter him from his commitment to Jesus. So as you continue this program, through any and all of your circumstances, don't allow anything to deter you from your commitment to Jesus.

2.3. What choices have you made concerning your commitment to this program? Think on Proverbs 16:3 as you contemplate this answer.

My personal prayer for all of you is that your commitment is 100 percent. Your attitude shapes the way you view your life and the way you view your progress in this program. Whatever personal trials or challenges you may face, set your thoughts on Jesus and the truth of his word, because this is your greatest source of encouragement and your strength. Never consider giving up.

2.4. What does Psalm 37:5 say about commitment?

"Commit thy ways unto the Lord, trust in him; and he shall bring it to pass" (Psalm 37:5). What this Psalm implies is simply to trust God and receive the benefits of his wisdom. Commit yourself to this program. Consider the many benefits to your life. Know that what you're doing is for the betterment of your life and your love ones. What you believe about God, his word, and yourself will determine your success. When you trust in God, he honors obedience.

2.5. Have you set a goal for this program? Is it realistic? Write your answer, then read Luke 14:28–30. What does this scripture mean to you?

"For which of you intending to build a tower, sitteth not down first and counteth the cost, whether he have sufficient to finish it"

(Luke 14:28). My response to your personal replies are with additional questions for you to think about:

1. What are your goals for this program?
2. Are they realistic?
3. Do you intend to achieve them?
4. Have you given any thought to what you'll be giving up to achieve your goals?
5. Is the cost to you worth it? Have you counted the cost?
6. Do you have the stamina or steadfastness to finish this program?

Think about these questions and write the answers in your book. Seven weeks is a long time, but a very short time for a lifestyle change and as a sacrifice for Christ.

2.6. Meditate on Ecclesiastics 3:1–9 and 2 Samuel 22:33.

Ecclesiastics addresses a time and a season for all things. How many of you have been putting off making changes in your life? What are some of your reasons or excuses? Has putting this off profited you anything? Are you better off for not putting your health first?

Think about your answers. This is your season. This is your time to be revived and renewed. This is the time to focus on your health. It's your season to make a lifestyle change. Let God be your strength in this endeavor. Meditate on 2 Samuel 22:33. "God is my strength and power: and he maketh my way perfect."

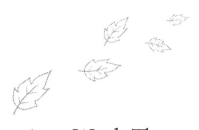

Revive Bible Study Discussion: Week Three

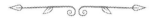

This is week three of the seven-week series of the Revive Bible study. Don't review this segment until you've completed your personal week-three Revive Bible lesson.

Week-three begins with vision, change, and transformation and Mental Secret Number Four: "Visualize success." Our premier scripture is taken from Habakkuk 2:2–3. A vision as defined in Webster's Dictionary is "the power of sight, the ability to see an image created in the imagination; a supernatural appearance." As we embrace this lesson, the need for and the importance of a vision for yourself will hopefully be revealed to you.

Questions and Discussion

3.1. Why do you think it's necessary to have a vision in mind when you begin this program?

You've been provided with a working definition for the term vision as taken from Webster's Dictionary. As you read question one and reflect on your thoughts and responses, I will discuss a vision and the importance of having a vision in mind when you begin this program. A vision is the ability to see change and transformation. It's the ability to see the end of something before it happens. The biblical definition of a vision is that it's a supernatural presentation of certain scenery or circumstances to the mind of a person either while awake or asleep. If this is true, your vision can manifest at any time. This is one reason why I encourage you to stay in prayer and spend time with God. This is also a reason that you should keep a pencil and notepad on your nightstand or bedside table.

Throughout the Bible, we constantly read scriptures of prophets and ordinary people who were shown a vision of what's to come. Isaiah, Ezekiel, and Nehemiah are just a few to see a vision of what's to come. Each saw—and here, I would like to quote Dr. Miles Monroe in his teachings of visions— "a clear conception of something that was not yet a reality but can exist."

Your vision should also be something that you clearly see but is not yet a reality, but which you clearly see can and will exist. It should be a strong image of your selective or foreseeable future. You need a vision for this program to keep you focused on what you want to accomplish. You need a vision for guidance and direction in your life. You need to see yourself as you want to be, not just in this program, but in every area of your life.

If you can't imagine or see where you want to be at the end of this program, then you may be stagnant and possibly just roaming aimlessly and endlessly. This is one of the reasons that you set a goal at the beginning of this program. If you haven't set a goal for yourself or this program, stop now and sit quietly, pray, and ask God for guidance.

3.2. Read Proverbs 29:18. Discuss its meaning as it relates to you and this program. Take the verses apart and analyze each.

This scripture emphasizes not only why you need a vision for this program, but also why you need a vision for the rest of your life. The scripture tells us that "where there is no vision [in essence, where there's no foresight, goal or direction, or just aimlessly wandering] the people perish."

Perish implies we die. We will leave this world not ever knowing what our purposes were. "But he that keepeth the law (God's law), happy is he." What is God's law as it relates to our bodies? Don't defile our bodies, because our bodies are God's temple. The end of this scripture says, "Happy is he." Why would you be happy if you stop defiling God's temple? How about freedom from chronic illness or obesity or just plain good health.

If you're completing the program individually, write your thoughts and review them in your private time. Take the time to rewrite and revise as new thoughts enter your mind. If you're completing the program with a partner or group. Take the time to discuss your answers openly. Keep the word of God in your heart and live by its principles. Stay in faith, and God will direct your path. This is your personal time with God and your personal, innermost thoughts. Be mindful about duplicating your materials for others.

3.3. Write your vision for this program. What do you see at the end of seven weeks? What do you see for the rest of your life?

As you write your vision for this program, take it a step further and clarify your vision in seven weeks. Take a leap and write down the vision for your life. As you write, remember: your vision is all about, and only about, you, no one else. It can't be for your children, husband, or anyone else. Whatever you write, just know that this is the vision you see for yourself and you can see the beginning and end before it actually exists.

3.4. Read Habakkuk 2:2–3. Separate each sentence. Meditate on each. How do these scriptures apply to you?

Let's apply the scriptures to what you've written. The scriptures say, "Write the vision down and make it plain upon the tables." How specific is your vision? Does it provide you with a vivid mental picture of what you want? "For the visions yet to come for an appointed time." How does this statement relate to the end of this program which is just four weeks away?

"Though it tarry, wait for it, because it will surely come." The vision will come quickly or slowly, depending on (1) the accuracy or clarity of what you've envisioned, (2) the intensity of your faith, what you're believing God for, and (3) your capability to guide your thoughts and activities toward your goal, which is changing your eating habits. We did not develop poor eating habits overnight, so they will not change overnight. But they will change if we keep working toward our goals.

3.5. Meditate on Philippians 4:13 and Philippians 1:6. Write your thoughts.

These are your personal thoughts. When you feel yourself getting a little delusional because maybe you can't see as much change as you would like, don't stop. Meditate on these scriptures and remember Philippians 1:6. "Be confident that he who has begun a good work in you will perform it until the day of Jesus." Working on being healthy and whole in everything and every part of your life is a good thing.

3.6. This is week number three; have you experienced change? This can be in your mind, body, or spirit. Write your changes, positive or negative. Next write what you want to improve and why?

Have you experienced change? Positive or negative. As you write your changes in this program, and in any other areas of your life, write what you want to improve and why. Only you know what your vision is. Just keep going, stay in the word of God. Keep your eyes on the prize—a heathier you.

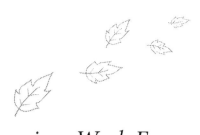

Revive Bible Study Discussion: Week Four

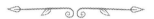

We are in week four of the seven-week series of the Revive Bible study. Don't review this segment until you've completed your personal week-four Revive Bible lesson.

Week-four Revive Bible study begins with discipline and Mental Secret Number Five: "Hold yourself accountable." Our premier scripture is taken from Genesis 3:12. "And the man said, the woman whom thou gaveth to be with me, she gave me of the tree and I did eat."

Questions and Discussion

4.1. What does accountability mean to you? Who are we ultimately accountable to? Read Romans 14:12. Complete your answers in the space provided.

Holding yourself accountable and taking responsibility for your own actions is a very important part in being successful in this program. When I think about accountability, I think about the definition used by three of the best-selling authors on accountability, Conner, Smith and Hickman in their book, *The Oz Principle*. "Accountability is a personal choice to rise above one's circumstances and demonstrate the ownership necessary for achieving desired results. To see it, to own it, to solve it and to do it." These are actions and words of wisdom that we should all live by. We as individuals make choices every day that affect our lives. Some are good and some not so good, but regardless of our choices, we need to take ownership and not cast the blame on others. Once we take ownership, we are free to direct our actions and thoughts toward achieving our goals.

Who are we ultimately accountable to? "So, then everyone of us shall give account of himself to God" (Romans 14:12).

4.2. Who is Adam blaming for his conduct or actions in Genesis 3:12? Why? Who should bear the blame for Adam's sin?

It appears that Adam is blaming his wife, Eve, because she listened to the serpent and disobeyed God. Adam should bear the blame for his sin. He, with knowledge of where the fruit came from, knowing that it was forbidden, took the fruit, and willingly ate it. He allowed something or someone to influence him. He willingly relinquished his right of free will, his right to make decisions in his best interest, to someone else. When we take our minds off the things of God and his word, we open our thoughts and actions to things that are not of God.

4.3. How can you apply accountability to this program?

You have choices in life. Are you making the best choices to succeed in this program, or are you blaming others for your lack of success? You have the power to take control of every area of your life including your health. You also have the power to control the lives and health of your children, those for whom you are responsible. Remember: the results of your actions are the direct results your choices.

4.4. Write as many words as you can think of that mean the same thing as the word *discipline.*

Discipline is being passionate. Where there's passion, there's consistency. Being consistent enables us to follow a chosen path or direction. This is one of the keys to success in any endeavor and the key to making a lifestyle change. View the list of words that you believe mean the same thing as discipline. If you have words such as *steadfast, endure, restraint, practice, self-control,* or many others, that's wonderful.

As I researched these synonyms for the word *discipline* from a biblical perspective, I discovered words such as *faithful, loyal, constant, staunch,* and *steadfast.* When I look at the term *faithful,* this implies an unwavering support or an adherence to a person, thing, oath, or promise. Our unwavering allegiance or devotion is to our heavenly father as we continue and complete this program.

Loyal implies a strong resistance to any temptation. This is a resistance to anything that will hinder you from the word of God and keep you from continuing to make a lifestyle change. *Constant* suggests or stresses a continuing firm or strict obedience to the word of God. Keep his word first and foremost as you complete this program. *Staunch* speaks of having the fortitude to be removed from influences that would weaken your resolve, or any attempt to sabotage your choice to serve God, and your choice to continue your lifestyle change. *Steadfast* implies a steady and unwavering allegiance to God and a firm commitment to this program. "Therefore, my beloved brother, be ye steadfast, unmovable, always abounding in the work of the Lord, for as much as ye know that your labor is not in vain in the Lord" (1 Corinthian 15:58). Your labor to make a lifestyle change is not in vain.

4.5. Read Job 36:10–11. In your own words, what do you think the scripture is saying and how can you apply it to this program?

One of Job's friends, Elihu, in this chapter is speaking out on God's behalf. He focuses on God's fairness, strength, and wisdom. He talks about how God teaches us his ways and outcomes, as Job continues to serves and obeys God. Verse 10 states that "he openeth also their ears to discipline and commandeth that they return from iniquity." When we are constant in the ways and word of God, and turn away from sin, we obey God. Verse 11 says, "We will spend our days in prosperity and our years in pleasure." As we open ourselves up to the knowledge of being healthy and discipline ourselves with our eating habits, we will spend our days in prosperity and health, and our years in pleasure. Obeying God and walking in his commandments grants us grace and favor; this includes our health.

4.6. Read Revelations 3:21. What does God promise to them that overcome?

"I grant to set with me in my throne, even as I also overcame, and am set down with my father in his throne" (Revelations 3:12). The scriptures speak to him who overcame the ills of this world and the sins of this world. These are the things that cause you to crucify yourself, the things that cause you to backslide. When you overcome these things, you, will the Lord allow to sit on his throne. Continue to be an overcomer with your health. And don't allow old eating habits to come back and contribute to ill health.

4.7. Read Job 11:14. What does the scripture tell us to do? How can you apply the scripture to this program?

"If iniquity (sin) be in thy hands, put it far away from you, and don't allow this wickedness to dwell in thy tabernacles" (Job 11:14). As we apply this to the program, you've begun a lifestyle change. This means your old eating habits, iniquity, or sin, is gone. You're no longer eating, for example, fried foods, white bread, white flour, white rice or cookies high in saturated fat. This is just to name a few. You're no longer eating junk food or sugary snacks. So, if this is in your house, get it out. This is temptation that causes us to sin if we submit to it. Don't allow anything or anyone to tempt you. Continue moving forward and always stay in prayer.

Revive Bible Study Discussion: Week Five

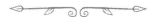

We are now entering week five of the seven-week series of the Revive Bible study.

Don't review this segment until you've completed your personal week five Revive Bible lesson.

Week-five Revive Bible study begins with perseverance and encouragement and Mental Secret Number Six: "Maintain a record."

Our premier scripture is taken from Proverbs 27:23 and 1 Thessalonians 5:11.

Proverbs 27:23 make reference to a shepherd's duty to know and maintain his or her flock in good condition so that the shepherd may reap the greatest value.

You're responsible for your health. You're the shepherds of your body. It's your duty to invest in, nurture and maintain your overall well-being by keeping a watchful eye to guard what goes in.

Keep a record of your daily physical activity, food intake, and liquids. Remove those things that are harmful that wreak havoc and cause ill health. Make sure to keep doctor's appointments, even if you feel great. If you do this, you'll reap the benefits of long life and prosperity. This is the greatest value.

Questions and Discussion

5.1. Write as many words as you can think of that are used in the Bible to mean the same thing as *perseverance*.

If you have words such as *constant*, *tenacity*, or *persistence*, you're on the right track. If you have other words, that's great also. *Perseverance* is a continuous or unceasing effort to achieve something that you've begun in spite of difficulties or hardships. It's also a constant persistence to a cause, action or purpose. Perseverance is an active key in every area of our lives. It's the key to our spiritual growth as you continue to seek God. It's the key to discovering your purpose, and it's the key to your success in this program. You must have a sincere desire to continue even when faced with adversities.

5.2. Read Hebrews 10:23. What do you sense God is saying to you?

"Let us hold fast to the profession of our faith without wavering for he is faithful that promised" (Hebrew 10:23). As you consider your thoughts, I will give you a few questions for consideration. As you continue in this program, do you have faith in what you're doing? Do you believe that you're improving your health, or are you questioning yourself? What are you asking God for? Trust him, believe in him, because God is faithful.

5.3. Read 1 Corinthians 3:14, then ask yourself what your personal reward is for continuing this program?

"If any man's work abides, which he hath built there upon, he shall receive a reward" (1 Corinthians 3:14). Here the apostle Paul is addressing building a strong foundation to the church of Corinth and stressing the quality of the materials used to endure and survive the trials. Your body is God's building. You bear responsibility for your contribution to its foundation and whether it will withstand the test of time. You're in week five. This is a clear indication that you're seeing results that you can build upon. This shows your commitment and sincere desire to make a lifestyle change. It also shows your commitment to God. Your personal reward to yourself for continuing this program is a stronger spiritual life and good health.

5.4. Rewrite your goals and expectations for this program. Next read Mark 11:24. Rewrite this scripture incorporating your goals into your personal prayer.

This question asks you to rewrite your goals and expectations for this program. Have your goals changed? What are your expectations now? You're also asked to read and rewrite Mark 11:24 into your personal prayer. As you pray this prayer, believe that God will give you the desires of your heart, if you believe without wavering.

5.5. How does your relationship with your mentoring partner indicate the kind of relationship you have with God?

5.6. Read Hebrews 10:24–25. How does this apply to your mentoring relationship? Write your answer, and next reaffirm your commitment to your mentoring partner.

Questions 5.5 and 5.6 addresses your relationship with your mentoring partner. Your mentoring relationship is personal between you and your partner. Make an effort to spend more time with your partner and with God. If you're taking the program in a group setting, share with your mentoring partner and reaffirm your commitment.

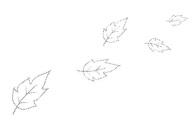

Revive Bible Study Discussion: Week Six

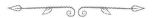

This is week six of the seven-week series of the Revive Bible study. Don't review this segment until you've completed your personal week-six Revive Bible lesson.

Week-six study begins with wisdom and knowledge and Mental Secret Number Seven: "Rebound and learn from your mistakes." Our premier scripture is taken from 2 Peter 1:2–3, 8. The key issue here is knowledge based on the word of God. Knowledge is ever growing. The more we grow in the knowledge of God the more we grow as healthy Christians.

Questions and Discussion

6.1. Read Proverbs 4:7, 22. How does God's word define wisdom? What does God' word say wisdom is to us? Underline the words, circle them, and engrave them in your memory. Next write your thoughts.

The scripture defines wisdom as "the principle of things and encourages us all to get wisdom and to get understanding." The scripture also says that wisdom is "light unto those that find them and health to all thy flesh." Another word for wisdom is *knowledge*. Knowledge is enlightenment. It's the ability to make use of what you've learned, to make correct decisions and follow the best course of action. It's the quality of being wise and following an established plan to gain a desired result. Throughout this program we have been learning and applying sound principles of nutrition and exercise, coupled with the word of God to aid us in living healthier and longer lives. As you continue this program, and after you've completed this program, continue to use the knowledge you've received to make wise decisions in all areas of your life.

6.2. Read Proverbs 4:10–11, 13 and John 8:32. What does God want you to learn, understand, and practice from these scriptures?

"Hear O my son and receive my sayings and the years of thy life shall be many. I have taught thee in the ways of wisdom; I have led thee in the right paths. Take fast hold of instructions; Let her not go; keep her for; she is thy life" (Proverbs 4:10–11, 13). Does it feel like God is speaking directly to you at this moment? He is literally speaking to you concerning your longevity. He is reminding you that, through his word, he has taught you and led you down the right path to health and long life. He wants you to learn and practice his ways and get rid of sin.

In just a short time, what we do know about this program is that it works. Our central focus is building your spiritual man and taming the flesh. If you can control this part of your life, you can, in most cases, control other areas of your life that may cause adversity. How many of you have lost the desire for some foods that are harmful to your health? How many of you have lost the desire to engage in behavior or activities that are unlike God?

6.3. Read James 4:7. This program is personal to you. Write your personal confession to God, then reaffirm your commitment to this program.

Submit yourselves to God and the things of God. Resist temptation in any form. This scripture reemphasizes your inability to excuse your conduct or your choice to engage in ungodly behavior. When you know what is right and you choose to do wrong, you're committing sin.

6.4. Read Colossian 2:21. Reword the scripture into your personal prayer.

You may choose to pray, for example, "Heavenly father, I thank you for your grace and mercy, I will touch not, taste not, or handle anything that may cause me to sin."

6.5. Read James 1:22, 25. What do these scriptures tell you, if you continue to be a doer of God's word?

The scriptures tell us that if we are doers of the word and not hearers only, we shall be blessed. in our deeds. If we continue in this lifestyle change, we will be blessed with good health and longevity.

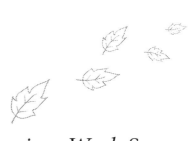

Revive Bible Study Discussion: Week Seven

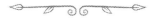

We are now in week seven, the final series of the Revive Bible study. Don't review this segment until you've completed your personal week-seven Revive Bible lesson.

Week-seven study begins with victory and revelation. Our premier scripture is taken from Matthew 25:21. "His Lord said unto him; well done, thou good and faithful servant; you have been faithful over a few things; I will make thee ruler over many things. Enter thou into the joy of the Lord."

Questions and Discussion

7.1. Why do you believe God led you to go through this program? Pray and meditate on this question, then write your answer. Read Proverbs 3:1–6.

As you meditate on the scriptures, receive the benefits of God's wisdom as you continue your journey of health and wellness.

"Come let us go up to the mountain of the Lord. He will teach us his ways so that we may walk in his path" (Micah 4:2). This scripture speaks to the restoration of the city of Zion in Jerusalem. Just as the scripture speaks of the restoration of the city of Zion, this program speaks to the restoration of your health by teaching you how to make lifestyle changes. Your answer to this question speaks to your relationship with God. Only through your walk with God will this answer be revealed.

God has prepared you for an assignment. Do you believe that you're moving to the next level in your spiritual walk? When you're faithful in small assignments, God gives you larger assignments. He has given you the keys to success and implores you to trust him and not forget his word.

7.2. Read Isaiah 40:5 and Philippians 2:13. Revisit question one and review your answer.

Isaiah speaks of Israel's deliverance from Assyria. God will pardon us from our sins if we will stop our past behavior and turn to him. The greatest success in the world is being obedient to the will of God. When you're obedient to God, his glory is revealed for the whole world to see, and this is what is happening to all of you. This program is not just about your health. It's also about your faith walk. It's about your belief and your trust in God. God is using you as a vessel to spread the good news of health and wellness. He has put you out there to show all that you come in contact with that this can be done and to show that you did not need pills or fad diets. "For it is God which worketh in you both to will and to do of his good pleasure" (Philippians 2:13). Continue to meditate on this scripture as you move forward.

7.3. Read John 16:13 and 1 Corinthians 2:9–10. Reflect on these scriptures in your private moments.

This is your faith walk with God. Take time to listen. He will tell you what is yet to come. At the end of this program you should have some idea as to what God wants you to do. Some of you may be fighting it, but it's there.

7.4. Only the spirit of God knows what God is doing in your life. Ask him what he wants you to do as a result of going through this program? Pray and wait on his answer.

As you wait on his answer, learn patience, because his timing is always right. Wait, expecting, but don't be in a hurry. Don't skip over your relationship with God. Wait and watch and see what happens. When you began this program, you started off thinking that this was all about the weight. You've since discovered that this program is about lifestyle changes in every area of your life. It's not just about the *weight*. It's about the *wait* on God. I sincerely pray that this program has been a blessing to all of you that participated.

References

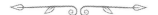

"About Fruits and Vegetables." *American Heart Association*. www.heart.org /HEARTORG/HealthyLiving/HealthyEating/Nutrition/About-Fruits-and-Vegetables_UCM_302057_Article.jsp#.WtTz5kxFxYc.

American Medical Association Family Medical Guide. John Wiley & Sons, 2004.

Balancing Carbs, Protein, and Fat, wa.kaiserpermanente.org/healthAnd Wellness?item=%2Fcommon%2FhealthAndWellness%2Fcond itions%2Fdiabetes%2FfoodBalancing.html.

Balch, Phyllis A. *Prescription for Nutritional Healing: The A-to-Z Guide to Supplements*. Avery, 2010.

Butler, Robert N. *The Longevity Prescription: The 8 Proven Keys to a Long, Healthy Life*. Avery, 2011.

Chan, Eric J., et al. "What Can We Expect from Omega-3 Fatty Acids?" *Cleveland Clinic Journal of Medicine*, 26 Feb. 2018, www.mdedge. com/ccjm/article/95072/preventive-care/what-can-we-expect-omega-3-fatty-acids.

Connors, Roger, Smith, Tom, Hickman. Tom. *The Oz Principle: Getting Results through Individual and Organizational Accountability*. Prentice Hall, 2004.

Daniels, Elsie Beauty Expert, Hollywood Faces 13 Jan. 2013

"Dietary Fats." *American Heart Association*, healthyforgood.heart.org/
eat-smart/articles/dietary-fats.

"Dietary Fiber." *MedlinePlus*, US National Library of Medicine, 1 Mar.
2018, medlineplus.gov/dietaryfiber.html.

Dietary Guide for Americans 2015–2020. Department of Agriculture,
Department of Health and Human Services.

Duyff, Roberta Larson. *Academy of Nutrition and Dietetics Complete
Food and Nutrition Guide*. Houghton Mifflin Harcourt, 2017.

"Eat Healthy Get Active" *American Cancer Society,* www.cancer.org/
healtheat-healthy get active

"Food and Portion Size." *American Diabetes Association*, www.diabetes.
org/food-and-fitness/weight-loss/food-and-portion-size.html.

"Good-for-You Carbohydrates." *American Cancer Society*, www.cancer.
org/latest-news/good-for-you-carbohydrates.html.

"Grains and Starchy Vegetables." *American Diabetes Association*, www.
diabetes.org/food-and-fitness/food/what-can-i-eat/making-healthy-
food-choices/grains-and-starchy-vegetables.html.

"High-Fiber Diet" *Pacific Beach Urgent Care, www.pburgentcare.
comhtml/high-fiber-diet.html*

The Holy Bible, King James Version.

Kowalski, Robert E. *The New 8-Week Cholesterol Cure: The Ultimate
Program for Preventing Heart Disease*. HarperCollins, 2002.

Mitchell, Marilyn, ND Natures Raw Truth 5 Oct. 2017

Munroe, Myles. *The Principles and Power of Vision: Keys to Achieving Personal and Corporate Destiny*. Whitaker House, 2003.

Price, Catherine. *Vitamania: Our Obsessive Quest for Nutritional Perfection*. Penguin Press, 2015.

Rosenfeld, Isadore. *Live Now, Age Later: Proven Ways to Slow Down the Clock*. Warner Books, 2000.

"Saturated Fat." *American Heart Association*, healthyforgood.heart.org/eat-smart/articles/saturated-fats.

Shandler, Nina. *Estrogen: The Natural Way*. Diane Pub Co, 1997.

Trickett, Shirley, and Karen Brody. *Candida: A Natural Approach*. Ulysses Press, 1999.

Twins Nutrition The, "4 Surprising Benefits of Vegetables." *CNN*, Cable News Network, 19 June 2014, www.cnn.com/2014/06/19/health/benefits-of-vegetables/index.html.

"Water: How Much Should You Drink Every Day?" *Mayo Clinic*, Mayo Foundation for Medical Education and Research, 6 Sept. 2017, www.mayoclinic.org/healthy-lifestyle/nutrition-and-healthy-eating/in-depth/water/art-20044256.

Watson, Brenda, and Leonard Smith. *The Fiber35 Diet: Nature's Ultimate Weight Loss Secret*. Free Press, 2007.

Webster, Merriam. *Webster's Dictionary*. G & C Merriam Co, 2008.

Weil, Andrew. *Natural Health, Natural Medicine: A Comprehensive Manual for Wellness and Self-Care*. Houghton Mifflin, 1995.

Xiao, and Chao Wu. "Health Effects of Soy Protein and Isoflavones in Humans." *The Journal of Nutrition* | Oxford Academic. *OUP*

Academic, Oxford University Press, 1 June 2008, academic.oup. com/jn/article/138/6/1244S/4670298.

Zelman, Kathleen M. "The Wonders of Water." *WebMD*, WebMD /a-to-z-guides/features/wonders-of-water#1.

Revive
The Wellness, Fitness and Beauty Program to Vibrant Health

To purchase this book online go to:
www.westbowpress.com
Search: D. McCants-Reed

To purchase this book by mail or the Instructor's
Guide visit: www.berevive.life

Printed in the United States
By Bookmasters